In Search
of Sleep

In Search
of Sleep

An Insomniac's Quest
to Understand the Science,
Psychology, and Culture
of Sleeplessness

BREGJE HOFSTEDE

Translation by
ALICE TETLEY-PAUL

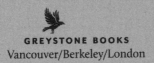

GREYSTONE BOOKS
Vancouver/Berkeley/London

First published in English by Greystone Books in 2023
Originally published in Dutch as *Slaap Vatten*,
copyright © 2021 Bregje Hofstede and Das Mag Publishers

Published by arrangement with Cossee Publishers
English translation copyright © 2023 by Alice Tetley-Paul

23 24 25 26 27   5 4 3 2 1

Permission for Gregory Orr, "Insomnia Song," in Lisa Russ Spaar (ed.),
Acquainted With the Night: Insomnia Poems (New York: Columbia
University Press, 2019) (p. 6) granted by the author.
Permission for "The Way" (p. 110) granted by the publisher.

Greystone Books Ltd.
greystonebooks.com

Cataloguing data available from Library and Archives Canada
ISBN 978-1-77840-016-2 (cloth)
ISBN 978-1-77840-017-9 (epub)

Editing for the English edition by Jennifer Croll
Proofreading by Jennifer Stewart
Jacket and text design by Belle Wuthrich
Jacket illustration by Blindspot/iStock

Printed and bound in Canada on FSC® certified paper at Friesens. The FSC® label
means that materials used for the product have been responsibly sourced.

Greystone Books thanks the Canada Council for the Arts, the British Columbia
Arts Council, the Province of British Columbia through the Book Publishing Tax
Credit, and the Government of Canada for supporting our publishing activities.

This book was published with the support of the Dutch Foundation for Literature.

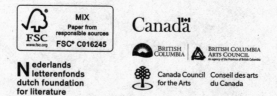

Greystone Books gratefully acknowledges the xʷməθkʷəy̓əm (Musqueam),
Sḵwx̱wú7mesh (Squamish), and səlilwətaɬ (Tsleil-Waututh) peoples on
whose land our Vancouver head office is located.

For Toine.
It's a beautiful day.

Is it me tossing
or is this bed
a small boat
in an unprotected
cove?
Haul
anchor, I suppose.
That is: turn on
a light and read
all night.

From "Insomnia Song,"
GREGORY ORR

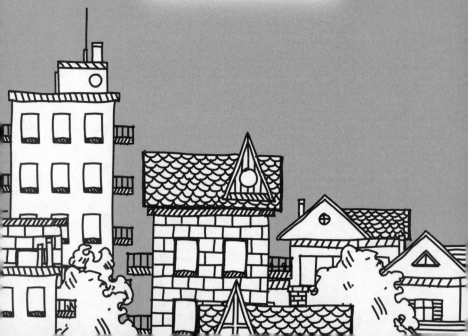

CONTENTS

00:00
Stargazing
11

THE BATTLE AGAINST SLEEP

01:00
All Animals Sleep
19

04:00
In Search of Sleep
32

02:00
Sleep as a Waste
of Time
21

05:00
Sleeping Pills
Don't Work
37

03:00
Sleep as
Performance
27

06:00
Desperately Trying
to Relax
42

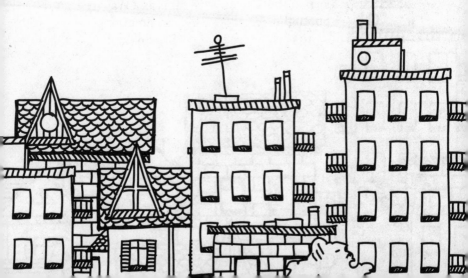

INSOMNIA IN THE BRAIN

07:00
We Don't Know
a Lot About Sleep
53

08:00
Sleep Isn't
Black and White
57

09:00
Hourglass
and Clock
66

10:00
Hyperarousal
70

11:00
The Bright Side
of Hyperarousal
73

12:00
Unprocessed
Emotions
80

13:00
Insomnia, Anxiety,
and Depression
83

14:00
Sleep and Mood
87

INSOMNIA AS AN ALARM

15:00
Insomnia Isn't
Simply a Defect
95

16:00
Sleep in the
Spotlight
103

17:00
You Feel More Than
You Feel You Do
109

18:00
Dreams as a Way to
Access Emotions
119

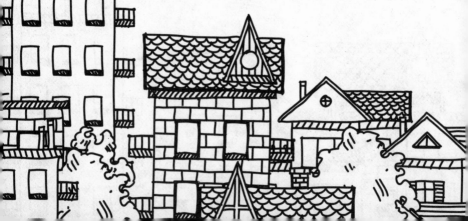

WHAT IS KEEPING YOU UP?

19:00
Context
135

22:00
Place
157

20:00
Money
138

23:00
Others
172

21:00
Time
151

00:00
The Weight of Sleep
189

ACKNOWLEDGEMENTS 201
NOTES 203
INDEX 247

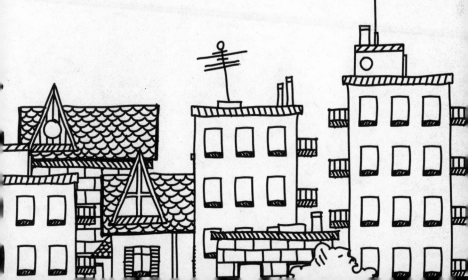

00:00
STARGAZING

I SAW THE MILKY WAY for the first time when I was eleven. It was a summer's night in the Peloponnese, a sparsely populated part of Greece, where I was on holiday with my family.

In the evening, after a day at the beach, we walked up the hill to a small ramshackle restaurant nestled between the olive groves. It was late, we were hungry, and the setting sun gave us legs like giraffes so we could reach the top more quickly. As we ate "Aunt Niki's" roast chicken, night crept up the hills. By the time we licked our fingers clean, our terrace between the olive trees had been transformed into an amber raft on a jet-black sea.

We switched on a flashlight and waded into the night.

It was a darker dark than I had ever experienced before. There was no one around, the bumpy road was unlit. The intense black enveloping us was so full of the sound of cicadas that it was as if the one were part of the other. Deafening darkness.

The bright beam of light that danced across the path in front of us illuminated my parents' footsteps, but shuffling along only a few paces behind them, we could barely see the ground under our feet. My sisters and I each demanded a turn with the flashlight and we took turns carrying it until, clumsily snatched and grabbed back, it fell on the path and went out.

We groped around for it. It was still warm from the extinguished light, like the cobbles, but it wouldn't turn on again. When the light's afterglow had disappeared from our retinas, it was as if the torchlight had crumbled and floated upwards. Countless stars appeared above us, and right in the middle was a white smudge.

My father forgot how annoyed he was about the broken flashlight and explained what we were seeing. That glittering band spanning the sky might look like a stripe, he said, but it is actually made up of hundreds of billions of stars. They are part of the Milky Way, the galaxy our sun also belongs to. It forms a huge spiral, and the stripe you see is part of it. The sun is one of the billions of stars in that spiral. And the earth is a small piece of rock rotating around that one star.

I struggled to believe what he said: that the Milky Way was always there, just you couldn't see it at home. It seemed crazy that something so incomprehensively big, which was also emitting light, could be hidden from view by streetlights, headlights, porch lighting. That something so trivial could make something so fundamental invisible.

I slept well back then. Without thinking. Sleeping was like breathing.

Twenty years later I was walking through Amsterdam one summer's evening. I was on my way to buy groceries, just before closing time. Mopeds buzzed past in the dirty-yellow dusk.

At the supermarket, I studied the brightly lit shelves for something to get me through the night. Yet again, I hadn't slept well in weeks. My eyes were dry from fatigue. I had read that eating something high in protein before bed could help. The more protein, the slower your digestion, and the less likely you are to wake up from a rumbling tummy. I didn't know if it was true, but I was willing to try anything.

I blinked as I read the labels.

Protein. Fat, saturated and unsaturated.

I was thirty and afraid of the night in a way I never had been as a child. I was looking for something to hold on to. Pills, powders, earplugs, bedtime tea, good habits. Each "solution" was a beam of light I followed until it went out, forcing me to go looking for something else.

That evening I bought Greek yogurt with extra protein: 12.5 grams per serving.

Somehow I knew I wouldn't find the solution to my insomnia in grams. Somehow I knew I was overlooking something. But I had no idea what else to do. I had tried every tip I could find.

I walked out with my purchase and didn't look up. There was never much to see between the streetlights. At most a moon, hardly any stars, definitely not the Milky Way.

I now know that about 40 percent of the global population never sees the Milky Way. There is too much light pollution. All sorts of things block our view of the stars: satellites, streetlights, the collective glare from all of our screens, lamps, and neon advertisements.

It irks some people. They set up groups such as the International Dark-Sky Association. They point out the negative effects of all that stray nocturnal light on various animals and claim the right to see the stars at night. Including the Milky Way, that fragment of the galaxy we are part of ourselves.

Essentially, they claim the right to see the bigger picture.

I slept badly for years. I spent most of my twenties engaged in trench warfare with the night, with any ground I gained being relinquished soon afterwards. It felt like it would never end. On bad days the fatigue was a wall I could barely peer overtop of.

Sleep became an interest, perhaps even an obsession. It was like I'd been dumped by a boyfriend I'd never cared much about—until he left, and I found out I couldn't live without him. And however much I tempted him, he wasn't coming back.

I only got over that insomnia when I accepted that my problem had nothing to do with *sleep*. Nor with the way I tackled sleep itself, with the practical elements of the night: bedtime tea, sleeping pills, my bedroom, with my "sleep hygiene" as I prepared for bed. I was focusing exclusively on the night, but the problem was the whole twenty-four-hour period: my days and how I spent them. Only when I started seeing my insomnia as a sign, an invitation to take a closer look at myself and see the larger context, did I work out how to navigate my nights again.

I learned to ask myself what was subconsciously bothering me so much that it was keeping me awake—that's what I had to do something about. It wasn't my nights that needed scrutinizing, but my days. Actually: my life. It's such an obvious insight I'm almost embarrassed to write it down. But still, this conclusion only became clear to me after puzzling over it for a long time, despite how much I read about sleep. It's a conclusion you rarely see others come to, because it doesn't fit into today's scientific outlook, with its preference for the neurological and mechanical. That outlook can teach us a lot about sleep, but it is incomplete. Chronic sleep problems are often not simply the result of poor sleep hygiene, so cannot be solved by some bedtime ritual or other, or a new mattress. Bad nights are the result of your days. And what's more, of the world in which those days take take place.

It took me almost a decade to work this out, and if some-one had told me ten years ago that I would have to reconsider all twenty-four hours of my daily life to be able to sleep at night, I wouldn't have believed them. That's why I'm pleased to share my journey with you.

In reality it took years; here I have condensed it into a single symbolic twenty-four-hour period. Those twenty-four hours start with a sleepless night, and the associated psychological battle with sleep. Then in the morning light of neuroscience I discuss the biology of lying awake. The afternoon marks a turning point: the insight that insomnia can be a signal that there's not something wrong in your brain, but in your life in more general terms. Finally I devote the evening hours to how to respond to that signal, by reconsidering how you relate to fundamental issues such as money, time, where you live, your ego, and the people around you.

If you have picked up this book, you are probably, like me, no stranger to the wee hours. A nice place to visit every now and then, on a night out with friends perhaps, but a hellhole if you are stuck there indefinitely on your own. You have probably, like me, tried anything and everything to sleep better—but still you lie awake. In that case, I invite you to follow me on my journey through the night. And to look further, beyond sleep hygiene. Because if I have learned one thing in all my restless nights, it's this: with sleep problems too, it is crucial to see the bigger picture.

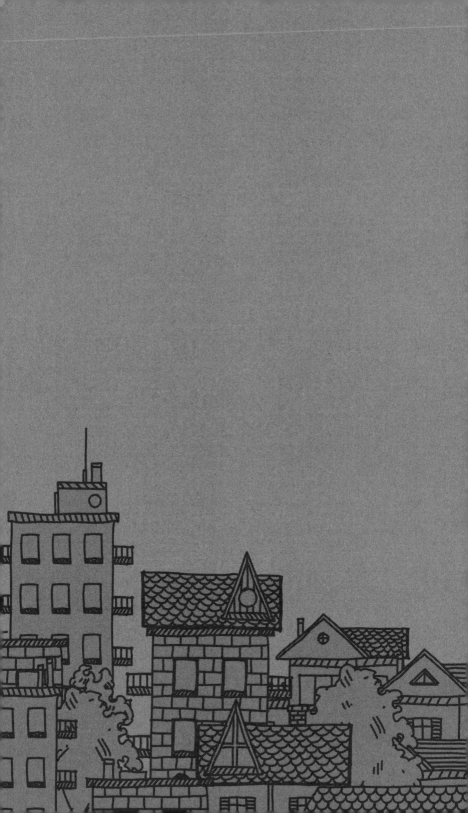

The Battle Against Sleep

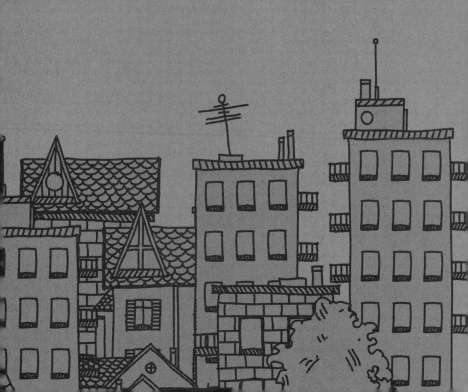

01:00
ALL ANIMALS SLEEP

WHEN I COULDN'T SLEEP, I would sometimes watch animal videos from the corner of the sofa in my room in Amsterdam.

Otters are my favorite. They float on their backs in the water, their paws folded across their chests; the fur on their tummies clumps together in wet strands. In pairs, they sleep holding hands so as not to drift apart. There is a clip of an otter floating on her back with her pup stretched out across her tummy. The pup is sleeping, rocked by its mother's breathing and the vast waterbed below.

I had to search a bit harder for sleeping elephant seals, but they were worth the effort. In the video, an elephant seal steers its two thousand kilos through dark blue water intersected by oblique stripes of splitting sunlight. As soon as it is deep enough—safe from killer whales and sharks—it turns onto its back, folds its hands across its tummy and motionlessly descends through the dark water. The voice-over calls it the "falling-leaf phase." After twirling down for fifteen minutes, the leaf becomes an animal again and starts moving, using powerful strokes to push its way back up for air.[1]

Some animals can sleep standing up. The flamingos at Artis Zoo, for example, which I often used to cycle past, sleep standing on one leg, with the other one buried in the warm down on their tummies.

In fact, there is no known species of animal that *doesn't* sleep. Even dolphins, which have to stay conscious to breathe, sleep with just one half of their brain, while the other half stays awake so they can continue to periodically surface and draw breath. Sleep is evidently so crucial that it finds a way.

Scientists believe that sleep must have come about with the first forms of life. It is an evolutionary constant that no species escapes. A spider tucks in its legs and its metabolism slows down. Earthworms assume a special sleeping position: slightly bent, like an ice-hockey stick. Even the simplest single-cell organisms have active and passive phases that correspond with the diurnal rhythm of our planet.[2]

However, for a great many people, sleep does *not* come automatically. If you join a supermarket lineup, one in five of the customers in front of you will have a sleeping problem.[3] In a class of secondary school students, half spend the night tossing and turning.[4] And about one in ten of us meet the strict clinical criteria for insomnia.[5]

If I could compete with the earthworm when it comes to sleep, I would never have written this book. If you could sleep easily, you probably wouldn't have picked it up.

In one way or another, human beings, the only animal species proven to have insomnia, made sleep complicated.[6] For example, by branding sleep as lost time: a temptation we shouldn't give in to.

If I really couldn't sleep, I would sink into the sofa, open up my laptop and say to myself: you know what, forget it. I'll do something useful instead. I'd sit there like that: grumpy and exhausted. Like a child who says, "I don't *want* to go to your stupid party anyway!"

02:00

SLEEP AS A
WASTE OF TIME

@elonmusk

the color orange is named after the fruit

I stared at this message, which appeared on my time-line without any context. It was followed by hundreds of responses, including:

@moment_in_time

Go to sleep lol

@yoboibleach

Elon what the Frick tis 3am and u tweet that does Elon ever sleep?

No, Elon never sleeps. The CEO of Tesla and founder of SpaceX is known not only for his ingenuity and his working pattern, but also for his inimitable nocturnal tweets. Fans regularly respond with the message: Elon, go to sleep.

But to the entrepreneur, sleep is a waste of time. In an interview with the *New York Times*, Musk said he regularly works 120-hour weeks and that his nights are usually a choice between "no sleep or Ambien," the well-known sleep-ing pill.[1]

People have been trying to master sleep for centuries, albeit in different ways. There was a time when Musk's attitude was the norm. In the nineteenth and twentieth centuries, for example, giving in to sleep was seen as a sign of weakness, while being able to stay awake was a desirable talent. There are still people today who don't pursue sleep, but instead view it with derision.

Donald Trump, for example, has been cultivating his "top dog" image for years, regarding sleep as way beneath him. He only sleeps for six hours a night. At least that's what he wrote in his first bestseller, *Trump: The Art of the Deal*. But that was in 1987. In 2004 he published a new book, *Trump: Think Like a Billionaire*, in which he claimed to sleep for a maximum of four hours a night. It only makes sense to sleep longer than that if you want to be insignificant, an "also-ran in life." In his latest book, *Think Big and Kick Ass in Business and Life*, Trump says he only needs three hours a night. (I am still waiting for him to announce he didn't sleep at all during his presidency.)

Because that's how passionate he is. According to Trump, "If you love what you're doing, you are probably not going to sleep more than three or four hours."[2] Tiredness is a motivation problem, at least if internet headlines are anything to go by: *These 7 Successful Entrepreneurs Almost Never Sleep. Five Bizarre Sleeping Habits of Successful People. How Much Sleep Do Millionaires Get? This Is How the Elite Count Sheep. How Many Hours Do Celebrities Sleep?*

Not many, if you believe the lists. Jack Dorsey (Twitter): four to six hours a night. Tom Ford (the fashion designer): three hours. Richard Branson (Virgin): five to six hours. Winston Churchill got by on four hours; Napoleon rarely slept any longer.

It is difficult to say how much people slept before modern times, but estimates suggest around seven hours.[3] Not quite the eight hours recommended by the World Health Organization, then. An idyllic time when people could sleep to their heart's content, undisturbed by work, noise, or pain, never existed. The idea that sleep is a waste of time isn't new either.[4] But it was the eighteenth century when people really started looking down on sleep. This wasn't a coincidence: the notion that a real man only needed four hours suited the demands of the Industrial Revolution. Those who had built expensive steam engines and factories could recoup their costs most quickly if they were running day and night. Cotton factories and iron forges were in production round the clock. That worked best if the people who kept them running worked as much as possible like the machines they operated: with an iron rhythm. The machines ran at all hours, and the alarm clock came into fashion to force sleep into a corresponding straitjacket.

It wasn't just factories that ran day and night; shops in big cities started staying open well past nightfall, setting in motion a change that gained further momentum around 1880 with the rise of the lightbulb. Wherever they flashed on, it suddenly became easy and affordable to banish darkness.[5]

In fact, the only thing still in the way of a perfect economic system was that strange habit people had of losing consciousness for hours each night. Couldn't we do something about that?[6]

The inventor of the lightbulb, Thomas Edison, thought we could. In the many interviews he gave during his lifetime, he was keen to state that people didn't need multiple hours of sleep at all. "A few minutes, or the occasional hour, is enough." And now he came to think of it, why did people still go to bed anyway? That habit had come about because people couldn't think of anything better to do with their time *before* his invention of the lightbulb. In the future, that absurd pastime would be a thing of the past. Sleep, according to the businessman, "is an absurdity, a bad habit. We can't suddenly throw off the thraldom of the habit, but we shall throw it off."[7]

Of course, he would stand to benefit from that. And he was not the only one with major interests in the ideal of the tireless employee. The longer the day, the more time to produce and consume. When the great inventor said that eighteen-hour working days should be introduced, the newspapers eagerly relayed that information.

Until well into the twentieth century, authors of popular self-help books also argued that sleep was useless and claimed you only needed very little of it. Two hours is plenty, they wrote. In his 1948 bestseller, *How to Stop Worrying and Start Living*, star author Dale Carnegie wrote that we have no idea how much sleep a person needs. "We don't even know if we have to sleep at all!"[8]

Over time, the amount we sleep has decreased globally, as has everything you can't make money from. According to the World Health Organization, on average we have relinquished a fifth of our sleep over the course of the last century. Back in 1998, the WHO warned that half of all adults in industrialized countries were suffering from disturbed sleep. The official recommendation is eight hours per night. Anything under seven is seen as "sleep deprivation," and harmful.[9]

However, around two-thirds of Dutch people sleep for seven hours or less per night. Almost a third get six hours or less.[10] Similarly, 65 percent of Americans sleep seven hours or less; 40 percent sleep just six hours or less.[11] In Britain, adults are losing out on a night's worth of sleep every week, averaging less than seven hours a night.[12] According to one poll, over half of U.K. adults sleep less than six hours per night; almost seven out of ten find their sleep is frequently disturbed.[13]

It's not only the nights that are fading away; the day-time nap is dying out too. In 2006, the Spanish government banned the siesta in governmental offices. The Japanese *inemuri*—a nap at one's desk, on a train, or wherever the mood strikes—is increasingly being rejected or even pro-hibited. In China, the right to a nap at lunchtime (*xiu xi*) was part of the constitution in 1950, but that right is also being eroded, and the break has been reduced from three hours to one.[14]

And that's why no office is complete without a coffee machine. The black drink—"the second-most-traded com-modity on the planet, after oil," according to sleep researcher Matthew Walker—ensures you no longer realize how tired you are.[15]

That doesn't mean your exhaustion has simply disap-peared. It is just hidden.

Imagine your head is an hourglass that starts filling up from the moment you wake. The fuller it gets, the more tired you are. The "sand" is actually adenosine: a chemical that accumulates in the brain with every waking hour. The more adenosine, the more you think: it's time for bed. The adenosine can only be broken down when you sleep. How-ever, if you don't get enough sleep, some of it remains for the start of the next day. That's why you need that coffee in the morning.

Caffeine makes you temporarily immune to adenosine. It blocks the receptors that are usually sensitive to it, so they cannot detect the adenosine still floating around in your brain and you do not realize (for a while) how tired you are. In the meantime, your hourglass continues to fill up and the "sleep pressure" rises.

Coffee does not resolve the tiredness, but merely conceals it. It's not just a drink—but one of the most popular drugs in the world.[16]

03:00
SLEEP AS PERFORMANCE

COFFEE CURES YOU from your sleep, Red Bull gives you wings, and you can sleep when you're dead. But the idea of sleep as wasted time is on its way out. Analyses and tests repeatedly show that short nights are bad for your health *and* for how you function. This has given rise to a stream of publications highlighting the importance of sleep, and the dangers of sleep deprivation.

Over the years in which my sleep deteriorated I noticed how the headlines changed: *Almost All Successful People Get Up Early* made way for *Sleep Your Way to Success. Sleep Powers Your Social Life*. And even: *Sleep or Die*.

While you once had to sleep as little as possible, now you have to get as much as you can.

I hear just how bad my sleeping pattern is for me when, after plowing through the headwind on my bike, I arrive at an office building not far from Amsterdam Central Station. I am met by Els van der Helm, a thirty-something sleep expert whose Dutch is peppered with English terms—a remainder from the time she spent at Harvard.

While the rain lashes at the windows, Van der Helm tells me, "Research in neuroscience is now able to show the effects of sleep deprivation very clearly." This type of research formed the basis of her PhD. "And those effects are truly dreadful."

"First, a broken night is detrimental to your reasoning, organizational, and problem-solving abilities. Those processes are all taken care of by your prefrontal cortex."

That's the part of your brain behind your forehead. The prefrontal cortex is one of the most recently evolved parts of the human brain. It enables us to carry out all sorts of complex tasks, such as planning and logical thinking. However, it is exceptionally sensitive to sleep deprivation. That soon takes its toll; after being awake for nineteen hours, you function as attentively as someone who has a blood alcohol content of 0.08 percent and is officially drunk.[1] Even that single hour's sleep we lose when we switch to Daylight Savings Time is reflected in a death spike the next day—mainly due to road traffic collisions.[2]

When you are sleep deprived, you probably don't even notice that anything is the matter, Van der Helm explains.

"In experiments where people are only allowed to sleep for four to six hours per night over a two-week period, they start making more and more mistakes in attention tests. At a certain point, their performance drops drastically. Yet still they keep saying: 'No, I'm fine.' You get used to your fatigue. After a while you forget how it feels to be properly rested." You might think that with enough coffee you are still functioning really well, but that might be because your judgment has been eroded by sleep deprivation.[3]

Logical thinking is not the only thing that takes a hit. After a bad night, you are less able to interpret social signals from other people. You also have the tendency to focus more on the negatives, and will remember those better than the positives, Van der Helm explains.

Your self-control goes out the window too. "People who don't get enough sleep display all sorts of compensatory behaviors. They might incessantly tap their foot, for example, to try and stay awake. And they eat more, drink more coffee, consume more sugar, and waste more time on social media," Van der Helm says.[4] I furtively think of the chocolate bars stuffed into my desk drawer.

"As I mentioned earlier, sleep deprivation weighs particularly heavily on your prefrontal cortex," she continues. "But that part of your brain is not only responsible for complex things like reasoning. It also has other important functions, such as keeping your emotional center, the amygdala, in check. If you have slept badly, you have a less effective 'brake' on your emotions, meaning you respond more impulsively and in a less controlled way." Various small studies suggest that test subjects kept awake spend more money the next day, mainly on junk food, and are more likely to make impulse purchases. Van der Helm also refers to research that suggests managers who slept badly are more impatient and irritable the next day, and more aggressive towards their subordinates.[5] I feel sorry for Elon Musk's colleagues.

The effects of too little sleep add up over time. Research shows that long-term sleep deprivation causes another important part of your brain, the hippocampus, to shrink (this is true at least for laboratory animals). That's bad news for our ability to learn, as the hippocampus is crucial for processing and storing information. That's why your capacity to learn new things is impaired if you don't get enough sleep.[6]

Your brain is not the only thing affected by sleep deprivation; your whole physical being suffers. Cardiovascular disease, diabetes, obesity, cancer, Alzheimer's, depression: every interrupted night is another ticket in that bleak lottery. Nurses who sometimes work night shifts, for example, are 60 percent more likely to get breast cancer. The more night shifts, the greater the risk.[7]

Depriving yourself of sleep is so harmful that the *Guinness World Records* no longer includes record attempts at staying awake. Skydiving from over 120,000 feet? Go for it! But sleep deprivation is seen as too dangerous.[8]

That's why sleep courses, awareness campaigns, and reports about sleep are forever springing up. Research agencies calculate the profit lost per employee that doesn't get enough sleep and is subsequently less productive due to absenteeism, health problems, accidents, or wavering concentration levels.[9]

Van der Helm also owns a company that offers sleep training aimed at increasing productivity. And there's a real call for her services. After all the recent articles and news reports about the disadvantages of sleep deprivation, the business world is starting to see that it's not longer days, but longer nights that are the key to superstar employees. Management companies recommend sleep as a "simple, easy, cheap way to boost productivity."[10]

In 1968, the year of the famous student protests in Paris, the following graffiti appeared along the route of the Paris Metro between the city center and the suburbs:

Vous dormez pour un patron.[11]

You sleep for a boss.

These days you might take that literally. Some companies already offer their employees a bonus for every night they get at least seven hours' sleep. They have to prove it by wearing sleep trackers, so their bosses can look over their shoulders while they're in bed.[12] In the Netherlands, the health insurer Menzis uses an app with trackers to offer a discount to anyone who scores "health points," including by getting enough sleep.

On the other hand, if you neglect your sleep you are fined. Elon Musk sparked protests when he gave that interview about his 120-hour working week. Investors sounded alarms about his mental well-being, and shares in Tesla fell by 9 percent.[13] The press called it unwise and irresponsible. Go to sleep, Elon, Twitter tweeted.

In fact, those who seek sleep fanatically have the same motivation as those who dodge it: to perform better. We once thought sleep took away the time in which to get everything done, but now we believe that a *lack* of sleep takes away the energy to do it. Whether you are seeking sleep or avoiding it, the aim is essentially the same: to get as much as possible out of the waking hours. Sleep as a step towards becoming superhuman.

And so sleep has become the umpteenth thing at which we can succeed. Or fail.

04:00
IN SEARCH
OF SLEEP

I'M NOT A FAN OF FAILING, and I'm even less a fan of being tired. So I diligently devoted myself to this new task. *Thou shalt sleep.*

Great, but how? I read up on it. I sifted through articles and books, such as Matthew Walker's *Why We Sleep*, an international bestseller about the importance of sleep. In it, he includes a deluge of studies revealing how bad it is for you to not get enough sleep. But he is an optimist; sleep is a matter of good habits. According to Walker, if you're not sleeping well, there's probably something wrong with your "sleep hygiene"—the way you prepare yourself for the night. His book therefore concludes with a list of tips designed to help. You probably know roughly what they are, since magazines and the internet are teeming with them. Don't smoke, don't drink. Don't drink coffee or have a big meal in the evening. Exercise, but not just before bed. Get some sunlight every day. Stick to a routine. Get black-out blinds. And a few others.

I took it all in. There came a time when I knew all the facts: that 65 degrees Fahrenheit is the ideal temperature for your bedroom; that it takes seven hours for your body to process half the caffeine in a cup of coffee; that the artificial light from lamps and screens can wreak havoc with your sleep cycle. And so on.

Not only did I know it; I also followed it to the letter. If good habits were key, great, I would adapt my habits. I got rid of coffee, then tea, then finally my beloved daily dose of dark chocolate. I bought blue light glasses and installed an app where a guy named Andy would tell me my legs were getting heavy.

There are a whole host of ways I tried to overcome my insomnia over the past years, in addition to the above.

More exercise.

Less sugar.

Eating something high in protein before bed.

A regular schedule.

A cool bedroom. A dark bedroom. A silent bedroom. Earplugs. Eye masks. Black curtains.

Meditating.

Not meditating, but simply going out with friends.

Working until my eyes stung. Stopping early and making time for an extensive sleep routine. A cup of warm milk, reading for an hour, a warm shower, lavender oil on the pillow.

Getting up if I couldn't sleep. Staying in bed if I couldn't sleep, not fleeing my bed, since what I am running away from becomes frightening in itself. Counting down from a thousand, in threes.

Writing down what I was thinking about. Dismissing everything I was thinking about as meaningless.

Cognitive behavioral therapy.

Melatonin. Magnesium. Valerian. Hops. Chamomile.

Smoking joints out the bedroom window until I was so high I could no longer stand upright.

And so on.

Despite my best efforts to improve my sleep hygiene, sleep remained elusive.

I decided more drastic measures were called for, whether or not they were legal.

A colleague told me she swore by THC, the psychoactive compound in cannabis. She discreetly got hold of a small glass bottle for me, filled with a dark-green, syrupy oil. A couple of hours before I went to bed that night I dripped a couple of drops under my tongue. The smell of rotting grass wafted through my nasal cavity; soon even my brain was filled with the smell of weed.

I thought of one of my former housemates, who was the best sleeper I'd ever known. You could find him on the sofa in our scruffy Brussels flat at any time of day, his head between the cushions, his legs dangling over the armrest. Every now and then he would get up to protect the cannabis plants in the garden from voracious slugs, although some days it was quite a task to outpace them.

I lay in bed expectantly. At first it was blissful. I could feel the muscles around my spine relax, like a series of locks being opened one by one: click, click, click.

I relaxed more. And more. I became so relaxed that it felt like I no longer had a spine.

Gradually the bones melted out of my body. I was no longer a woman relaxing in bed, I was no longer a woman. I seriously started to think I had turned into a slug. Maybe have a quick look? Opening my eyes would be helpful, but that no longer seemed to work. Did I even have eyes still? Perhaps I would have to push them out on stalks through the blubber of my body. Having pondered my metamorphosis for a while, I decided I didn't want to be a mollusk. I tried shouting for help, but that no longer worked either. Slugs don't shout. Thankfully, I finally fell asleep.

It was a suffocating experience, and the lethargy of the slug-woman lingered for the next two days. I decided that was enough experimenting, but I soon forgot those good intentions when the pressure became too high.

One night I was staying on a friend's sofa. Her black cat, unhappy about the intruder in its spot, tiptoed back and forth over the backrest. It kept at it for a long time before finally sitting down, its eyes still fixed on me. Every now and then I would look up and see the green membrane behind its eyes glowing in the reflection of the streetlights. I started feeling more and more uneasy. After all, cats are predators, I thought. I could feel my throat tightening. My nose blocked up too, and breathing became a struggle. When my friend finally came to investigate the wheezing sound, she got a shock when she saw my swollen head, and quickly gave me some antihistamines.

That's how I discovered that not only am I allergic to cats, but also that antihistamines make me very sluggish. So sluggish that they send me to sleep.

I took them for a while, even when there weren't any cats around. But the adverse effects were too great; the associated sluggishness lingered all day. If I was going to feel that groggy anyway, I decided I may as well take a less silly route to the same result: getting up at night and doing something.

I took a phased approach. First, I would *threaten* to get up, the way you pretend you're walking away from an argument, hoping you'll be called back again. I would go to the toilet and then come back again, hoping for a type of "reset," a new chance.

If I still wasn't asleep after three trips to the toilet, I would get up again, put on my dressing gown and go to the kitchen. I would try to avoid looking at the red digits on the microwave clock as I spread peanut butter onto a rice cake, making sure it went right to the edges and there weren't any clumps. I would eat it standing by the kitchen window, in the glow of the traffic lights outside, which would keep jumping from red to green.

The next step was distraction. I would read something, or switch my phone on and search for sleeping animals.

Birds have a wonderful way of doing it. When a flock perches on a power line to rest, all of the birds fall into a deep sleep, except for the first and last ones. They each keep one of their eyes open, the outer eye in the line. Those two birds use one eye and one half of their brain to monitor their environment, while the other half of their brain sleeps. After a while, those outermost birds on guard duty turn around so as to keep watch with their other eye and the other half of their brain. The flock behaves like a single creature that always keeps two eyes open. Sleep is not something for the individual, but a process that the whole group takes part in.[1]

I sometimes wonder whether that used to be the case for people, and if that's why some of us sleep more lightly than others today.

05:00
SLEEPING PILLS DON'T WORK

IN THE CITY, you can't always tell when dawn arrives. It never gets dark. But at some point the pale-yellow light changes, and it becomes cooler and bluer.

If I was still awake at that time, I would start my day. I'd throw on a big hoodie and sink into the corner of the sofa with a strong cup of tea and my laptop, and continue working on an article or novel.

It was a relief to focus on something else, and funnily enough it worked well too. Insomnia doesn't make me drowsy. Instead of being in a haze, on days like that there is a taut focus that only occasionally rips, revealing the fatigue underneath. I got through those days pretty well, but that was all. I was merely functioning; I didn't have the energy for any flourishes.

When I finally contacted my doctor, she prescribed me temazepam. I didn't really want sleeping pills as I was concerned about addiction and side effects (more on that later). But I didn't see many other options.

For a while the pill beside my bed served as a white emergency button. It reassured me that I had the choice to avoid the lonely hours, and that I could escape the panic that lapped at my mind like the tide at a sandcastle. Just a couple more nights like that, I would think, and I will go crazy. The strip of tablets hushed: if you really can't sleep, at least you can pass out.

The dose needed for that gradually increased. At first, half a tablet was enough, but before long a whole tablet wouldn't cut it. I would often lie half-awake in bed with the metallic taste of the sleeping pill on the back of my tongue. It was a strange in-between world; I was no longer awake, but the state I found myself in couldn't be described as *sleep* either. I could hear what was going on in the house, for example, but couldn't make sense of the sounds, as if each thought was instantly paralyzed. I couldn't fully slip away from the world. My mind was compressed like the trash in a garbage truck, but there was always a crack of light, a sliver of consciousness that refused to let go. And in the mornings, the chemical hangover got worse and worse.

One in ten Dutch people use tranquilizers or sedatives. And these are just benzodiazepines, such as oxazepam and temazepam—not even counting Z-drugs like zolpidem (Ambien). Since the Dutch government started actively discouraging people from taking benzodiazepines, use has fallen somewhat, but in 2017, 161.5 million defined daily doses were dispensed.[1] Let that sink in for a moment: 161 million tablets. In the Netherlands alone. In one year.

And one finds comparable figures elsewhere. In the USA, 12.6 percent of adults use benzodiazepines, meaning roughly one in eight,[2] while use among young adults has soared.[3] One in ten Canadians takes prescription sedatives; this figure is even higher among seniors.[4] It's hard to get clear numbers, because misuse of these drugs (meaning use without prescription) is considerable.[5]

What do sleeping pills actually do? I contacted neuroscientist Eus van Someren to find out. Van Someren is a small, energetic man with unruly hair and a boyish face, despite the wrinkles. He is the head of the Sleep and Cognition department at the Dutch Brain Institute and a professor of integrative neurophysiology. He talks about sleep with an infectious enthusiasm.

"Sleeping pills such as temazepam and zopiclone act on a specific neurotransmitter in your brain, known as GABA. GABA suppresses communication in your brain. Sleeping pills reinforce its effect," he explains.[6] You can think of GABA as your body's own sedative. It prevents signals from being passed on in your brain, in other words preventing you from noticing things. "What it means is that you no longer *realize* that you aren't sleeping. Sleeping pills shouldn't be called sleeping medication, but anti-wake medication instead. Pills like that certainly do something, because if you take a couple, no one will claim that you are *awake*. However, they don't give you the kind of sleep you would normally get." Sleeping medication cannot simply induce natural sleep, Van Someren explains. No medication can do that. And unfortunately the "artificial sleep" they provide fails to create the healthy, restorative effect of real sleep.

Other sleep experts also warn that sleeping pills aren't the answer. In *Why We Sleep*, for example, Matthew Walker states that while some modern pills like Ambien produce something akin to sleep in terms of brainwaves, they do not succeed in inducing real sleep. The result lacks the slow brainwaves that occur in natural sleep. And above all, it lacks the regenerative effect.

So there are not many advantages, but plenty of disadvantages. Memory loss is one of them. Whereas sleep strengthens your memory, sleeping medications lead to forgetfulness. That's because sleep reinforces the connections between brain cells, whereas sleeping medications weaken them.

If that doesn't make sleeping pills unappealing enough, there's also a good chance that all they are doing, at best, is delaying your insomnia. As soon as you stop taking them, you can suffer from what's known as rebound insomnia: worsened sleep caused by the withdrawal. As a result, you are more tempted to reach for the pills and end up caught in a vicious circle. Even if you accept that, there is not much magic left in them once you learn that people who take pills sleep barely any longer than they would without them.

People today find it difficult to accept that sleep can't be forced. We can create embryos, grow hamburgers in a petri dish, produce fluorescent rabbits, change the climate of a whole planet. However, despite all the research, pills, and efforts, there is not a single way to induce or replace sleep.

When a team of researchers reviewed 65 different studies into the use of sleeping pills, they found that those who took them barely slept any better and didn't fall asleep any more quickly than those given a placebo. The people given a real pill fell asleep 22 minutes sooner on average. What's more, that effect was mainly apparent in the older studies, when pills contained higher doses. All in all, the researchers concluded that the clinical effect of sleeping pills is "rather small" and their clinical significance "questionable."[7] They do something, but the same can be said for a placebo. Furthermore, a psychotherapeutic approach works just as well as pills in the short term, and better in the long term.[8]

On the other hand, sleeping pills—unlike placebos or a visit to the psychologist—have undesired side effects, such as potential addiction. In addition, they often leave you feeling groggy the next day, increasing the likelihood of you ending up in a traffic accident or getting injured in a fall. That's just one of the reasons why users of sleeping pills are at greater risk of dying than the average person. The suspected link between the pills and cancer is another factor; those who take sleeping pills have a 35 percent greater chance of getting cancer.[9]

If you know these things, it is crazy to think that we are taking so many pills that are giving us side effects, but no sleep.

06:00
DESPERATELY
TRYING TO RELAX

I DITCHED THE PILLS. It was time for real help. I wheeled my bike to my appointment. The wind sent leaves flying up into the air, bare branches tapped against each other. I was lightheaded and my body was so wispy I could barely feel my legs move. If I didn't hold on to my handlebars, I would be swept away.

At the end of the appointment, the psychologist assessing my case said, "It's up to you. I can either assign you a sleep disorder or an anxiety disorder. Because you're anxious about not being able to sleep, you meet the criteria for both perfectly." She slid the questionnaire I had filled in towards the middle of the desk and put her hands on top of it. A golden ring with a gemstone in it. Even her fingers were freckled. She looked at me cheerfully, her whole face and neck covered in sunspots.

I don't like being labelled as disordered. Now it's up to me: disordered in general, or just in bed?

"Does it make a difference for the treatment?"

She shrugged. "Well, for a sleep disorder I can prescribe you standard sleep therapy. If you go with an anxiety disorder, you have more options. I can send you to a sleep therapist who has a broader approach."

"Okay. I'll do that then."

As she turned to her screen, I closed the notebook I'd brought with the long list of figures in the back. Two, three, five, eight, two. I had been keeping a record of how many hours' sleep I got each night for months. I had prepared myself for a diagnosis and with it the right to assistance, but succeeding with these figures didn't feel very triumphant.

"Gen-er-al-ized-anx-i-ety-dis-or-der," the psychologist mumbled as she entered her diagnosis into my file. A decisive tap on *enter*. "Right! You will get a phone call in due course to arrange an initial consultation."

And with that I was back outside again.

You can choose? Is that how it works?

I walked back the same way I had come, retracing my steps through the park. A lime-green bird flew overhead, into the crosswind. Wide wings, a long, pointed tail, a shrill laugh.

A couple of weeks after my referral I got a call for my initial appointment with the sleep therapist.

Red brick, small balconies, bikes outside. A discreet sign by the door indicated I had found my way to Grip Psychologists. I rang the bell, descended a flight of stairs and was let in.

Half of the treatment room in the basement was set up as an office, with a big desk and a whiteboard. The other half was arranged like a living room, with sheepskins draped over tub chairs I would never sit in over the months I came here. A skinny Swiss cheese plant by the window raised its branches towards the light.[1]

The therapist sitting opposite me was Sanne Verkooijen, a young woman with a serious expression who wore her straight brown hair draped over her left shoulder. She asked me to tell her all about my attempts to sleep. She noted everything I summarized on the whiteboard behind her desk. Over the next fifteen minutes, her squeaking blue marker sketched out my entire daily life: what I ate, when I showered, worked, exercised, met up with people or not, what temperature the thermostat was set to. She wrote down all my futile practices, including the rice cakes with peanut butter. Insomnia as a full-time job.

"And, does it work?"

I snorted. I'm not crazy, I could see my desperate attempts to get some sleep weren't helping. But the longer the insomnia went on, the more willing I was to try anything.

She asked me if I could remember a time when I did sleep well. "As a child, for example?"

Yes, as a child. I remember waking up one New Year's Day in my grandparents' attic and realizing I had missed the countdown to the new year. They had promised they would wake me up for the fireworks, but now it was suddenly the next day! I was so angry. "We couldn't wake you," Granny and Grandad said. "Not even with a wet flannel in your face."

That same grandad took me and my sisters on a skiing holiday. The first highlight of that holiday was the sleeper train, which took us as far as Italy. It was an old, gray beast with indestructible plumbing, mustard-colored curtains, and erratic heating. We excitedly took possession of our carriage, with space for six beds. It was a world unto itself, with a small ladder, moving furniture, a long, swaying corridor... I was allowed one of the top bunks: a fabric-covered plank right under the roof, a good six feet above the ground. Because of the height, it sloped towards the wall, so you were more likely to roll into the wall than out of bed. There was also a net that could be stretched out between the two top beds. If you were to tumble out of your bunk in the night, you would fall into that net. The protection it offered was mainly symbolic: the net was barely big enough for a six- or seven-year-old, and every time I "accidentally" rolled onto it, it creaked ominously. But it was safe in my mind.

And I slept. Despite the announcements at the stations, despite the skiers and snowboarders who bashed their skis and suitcases into the sliding doors at every stop, and despite how much the train shook as it labored up the hills.

Sleep was once a god: Morpheus, the god of dreams. In paintings, he is a handsome winged youth who takes the sleeper in his arms. My father sometimes refers to him when he's in a poetic mood. "I'm going to crawl into Morpheus's arms for a moment," he says when he treats himself to a nap.

Morpheus has long since retired, like all the gods. He was replaced for a while by the far less formidable Sandman, a gnome-like character found in European folklore with a pouch of sand on his belt. He would sprinkle it onto your face and you would fall asleep. You never caught him in the act because he would only come if your eyes were closed— and the only trace he would leave behind was the yellowish grit you rubbed out of your eyes in the morning.

As a child I could easily surrender to sleep. I trusted a flimsy net, and even an invisible gnome. When I grew up, it no longer worked.

The only thing that could really comfort me twenty years later was the weight of my boyfriend. When we spent the night together, on a bad night I would sometimes ask him, "Can you squash me?" He would then roll over from his side of the bed and sprawl out on top of me. The aim was for him to cover as much of me as possible, his legs on my legs, his tummy on my back, his arms on mine, so that I was pushed into the mattress so firmly that only my hands and feet could move.

Strangely enough, it was wonderful. His 150 pounds of inescapable presence brought me to a standstill, pushed all the restlessness out of my body. All the air too, incidentally. After a couple of minutes I would have a fit of laughter, gasp for air, and my boyfriend would have to get off. Then he'd roll over again, grumbling, "What a unique specimen I've got here."

Sometimes I would then fall asleep. Other times I wouldn't. But the racing of my mind had at least been curbed for a moment.

When I told the therapist about the sleeper train and the Sandman, she said, "It sounds like sleep was automatic at one point. Like you could easily surrender to it."

Yes, it was at one point. But surrendering later became something I had to force.

Pointing to the whiteboard filled with all of my attempts to sleep, she said, "Sleep is the ultimate form of relaxation, which is ironic because desperately trying to relax will only backfire."

Daily run, I read; *no tea or coffee*; *counting down from a thousand*. Desperately trying to relax will only backfire.

"There's nothing you can do to achieve the ultimate form of doing nothing. On the contrary, if you are trying so desperately, sleep becomes something you are battling: an enemy you have to defeat with herbal tea and meditation.

If that's your attitude, your stress system springs into action, the same way it would in any battle."

Verkooijen explained that many people who ended up in this treatment room had started seeing sleep as something to struggle with—an enemy, actually. "The characteristic I notice time and time again among people with sleep problems is a need for control. It's often young people—mainly women—who want everything all at once: a family, a perfect home, to excel at work, to exercise, to keep seeing their friends... All of those wants make your brain incredibly active."[2]

People subsequently apply their need for control to their sleep.

It doesn't help that we live in a society in which anything is possible, Verkooijen added. If you are used to life going your way if you just put some effort in, you expect sleep to work the same way. As long as you take the right steps, you expect sleep to follow automatically, like a sticker on your neat homework. But no. There's nothing you can do to achieve the ultimate form of doing nothing.

"Look," my therapist said, walking up to the whiteboard and drawing a big dot on it. "This is your original problem: you can't sleep. And these"—she drew a circle around the dot—"these are all the things you have built up around it in an attempt to sleep. The more of these you add, the bigger the problem becomes. It simply keeps growing until it consumes your whole day. And as a result, it becomes even more difficult to switch off at night."

She paused for a moment, as if for effect, and let me take in the dot and the circle, which stared back at me like an eye. "That's why it's better to stop all your endeavors to get your sleep back on track. Or: if you want to reduce your sleep problems, don't do anything about them."

Don't do anything. Nothing at all. "Let go," she said. So that's what I'd gone to Grip Psychologists for.

Did that mean I could do everything again with impunity and it wouldn't matter? Goodbye meditation, chamomile tea, and exercise. Hello blue light, coffee, and wine on the sofa.

It was scary to let go of all the things I depended on, however hopeless they were, yet at the same time it was also liberating. Shortly after my conversation with the sleep therapist, my friend and I went to the cinema to watch a thriller, which we discussed afterwards in a café. Then—so late, so contrary to my routine!—I walked home through a rain-soaked city, where all the lights appeared double because they were reflected on the wet stones. It was after midnight by the time I got to bed, with a head full of experiences and alcohol, and I slept badly, as usual, but at least I'd had a good time.

I was relieved, but also disappointed. If your whole being is in dire need of sleep, that necessity doesn't suddenly disappear, and doing nothing on doctor's orders is hard to digest.

I settled for a compromise. If I couldn't do anything to physically get sleep, I could at least try to understand it. I wanted to find out why all my tidy, sleep-friendly habits were so clearly in vain. If sleep hygiene wasn't the solution and therefore wasn't the problem either, was there perhaps another reason why I was lying awake?

Searching for an explanation for my insomnia was, of course, cheating. It was a way of getting round not doing anything: a shortcut to a possible solution, while the therapist said that I should forget the idea. But hope dies hard, and I am stubborn.

There was also another reason why I wanted to search for an understanding of sleep. The thing I hated most about my insomnia was that it seemed so pointless. I can put up with a bit of discomfort as long as it serves a purpose. (Getting up at four in the morning to go on holiday feels completely different from getting up at four in the morning because you just can't sleep.) It seemed to me that lying awake would be easier if it had some sort of meaning.

And that's how, after almost ten years of insomnia, I started a project: to read everything and speak to anyone who could explain my insomnia to me.

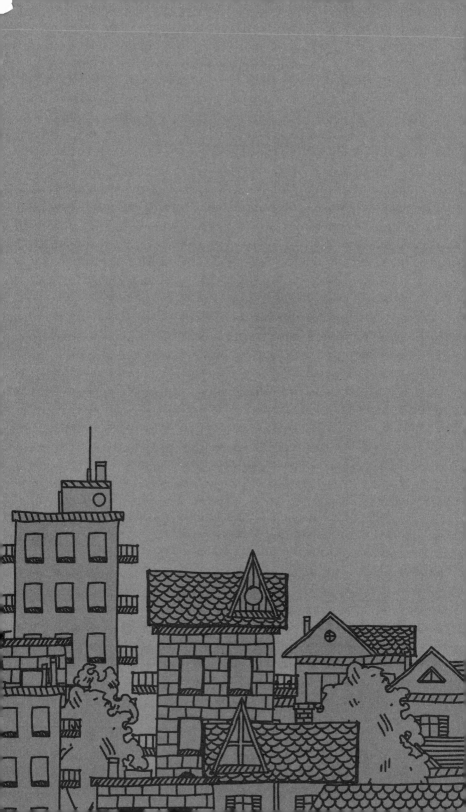

Insomnia
in the Brain

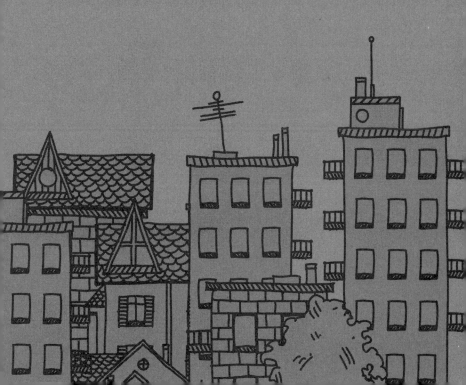

07:00
WE DON'T KNOW
A LOT ABOUT SLEEP

IF YOU START LOOKING into the meaning of insomnia, it won't be long before you encounter the first obstacle: according to many good sleepers, insomnia doesn't exist.

If you claim you sleep badly, you are perhaps familiar with the cheerful response, "Oh, you're getting more sleep than you think." One of the most stubborn myths about insomnia is that it's all in your head. You just *think* you're lying awake. There is a term for it—sleep state misperception—and therefore it must be true.[1] Insomniacs are wrong. Their nights are actually great.

In his bestseller, Matthew Walker even states that most insomniacs are simply hypochondriacs. That's because if you get these people to spend the night in a laboratory, and stick electrodes that measure sleep "objectively" all over their heads, the equipment often contradicts what the people themselves are experiencing: that they are sleeping really badly. The sleep graphs the computers churn out reliably show brainwaves associated with sleep, even those associated with deep sleep. They may be interrupted, but if you put all those chunks of sleep together, the test subject had a decent night's sleep, even though they claim they were lying awake for hours.

How do you determine whether someone is lying awake? It was the first question I had to answer, and that proved rather tricky.

Sleep is perhaps a universal part of life, but despite its ordinariness it remains surprisingly mysterious. We don't actually know a lot about sleep. What is it, why do we do it, how does it work, and why does it go wrong? We have, at best, smart hypotheses.

What happens when you are asleep? How does it feel, how does it work? It is impossible to say. You can't study your own sleep—after all, you are *asleep* at that moment. You can only access someone else's sleep via a detour too: through their vague accounts after waking, by looking in from outside, or from readings taken from an inaccessible brain, which you then translate into colorful images or graphs.

Maybe you have found yourself discussing whether or not you dozed off when you had a quick lie-down on the sofa. No, you think, you still heard everything, and you were thinking about a problem at work. Yes, you were asleep, the person sitting next to you maintains: she heard you snoring gently, and a dribble of saliva on the cushion seems to prove her right.

A sleep graph called an electroencephalogram (EEG) is used to establish what is classed as sleep in scientific terms. But that already presents the first problem, Eus van Someren explained. I introduced him earlier: a boyish man with unruly hair; head of the Sleep and Cognition department at the Dutch Brain Institute. He taught me more than anyone else about sleep, so he will come up quite a bit in the following chapters.

Van Someren explains that the notion that insomniacs are making up their condition really bothers him. He says, "People who say that always use sleep graphs as their proof. But what they are forgetting is that an electrical signal like that doesn't measure very much at all." On an EEG, he explains, you can see how many electrical signals are recorded in the brain while someone is asleep. Those signals are translated into a wavy line; and some of these waves are characteristic of sleep. But what do those waves actually mean? Van Someren explains, "A brain wave shows that many brain cells are changing activity at the same time. But this is not an exact measurement: you only see something when between 50,000 and 100,000 brain cells are changing activity at the same time. If fewer than that are changing activity, it won't pick that up." In other words, an EEG only measures general changes. "Furthermore, the electrodes you stick onto a person's head to measure these waves only measure what is going on in the *outermost* layer of the brain, the cerebral cortex. They don't register what is going on deeper inside," he explains.

"It's a bit like this: you've got a big, old-fashioned computer, which you have been putting through its paces. Then at some point the fan comes on, and you can hear it buzzing. You can think of our brain as that computer. And the buzzing of the fan is the EEG: it tells you that there's a lot going on in that computer, or in that brain. But you have no idea *what's* going on. You can derive something from the EEG, but it's maybe only 0.1 percent of what's happening in the brain. In all honestly, I think it's much lower than that. I think almost everything remains under the radar."

In other words, electrodes and sleep graphs only reveal a fraction of what is going on in the cerebral cortex, the outermost layer of the brain. By far most of what is going on in the brain remains hidden.

These words from one of the Netherlands' leading sleep researchers don't seem a very promising start to my search for sleep. The more I learn, the clearer it becomes that sleep is more complex than I had thought. It seems to be a field that is still mainly in the dark and about which there are still many questions.

In the coming chapters we will delve into those parts of sleep over which science *has* already cast its morning light.

08:00
SLEEP ISN'T
BLACK AND WHITE

WE OFTEN THINK of sleep as an on-off switch: you are either awake, or you are asleep and out for the count. But that's not how sleep works. Drawing a clear line between being awake and being asleep proves difficult. Instead, there are all sorts of intermediate stages. Rather than a swimming pool you dive headfirst into, sleep is like surf; the waves engulf you in one moment, and then only splash you with spray and foam the next.

Sleep isn't black and white in the way it is structured, either: it occurs in various phases, with some resembling wakefulness more than others.

The best-known sleep phases are dream sleep and deep sleep, also known as REM sleep and NREM sleep respectively.

REM stands for rapid eye movement. You might have observed someone who has dozed off beside you on the train, and noticed how their eyes appeared to flit back and forth behind closed eyelids: this is rapid eye movement.

But those moving eyes are not the only characteristic of REM. REM is also a lighter phase of sleep from which you can easily wake up. Furthermore, if you wake someone up during REM sleep, they are likely to tell you they were in the middle of a dream, which they can relay to you in living color. That's why REM sleep is often called "dream sleep."

REM sleep has another name too: paradoxical sleep. The paradox is that the REM brainwaves you see on a sleep graph are very similar to the waves recorded from an awake brain. An awake brain and a brain in REM sleep both produce chaotic scribbles. These scribbles indicate that various parts of your brain, at the time of the recording, are processing all sorts of information simultaneously: smells, sounds, feelings ... That doesn't produce a neat pattern, but a jumble. This is the same whether someone is awake or whether they are in dream sleep.

The fact that the EEG doesn't show much of a difference between REM sleep and being awake means that it is very difficult to differentiate between them on a sleep graph. That's why an EEG is not capable of officially determining whether or not someone is asleep; their body must, for example, also be limp before sleep scientists can draw such conclusions.[1]

Furthermore, what may look like sleep to an outsider often feels very different to the sleeper, Van Someren explains. "If you wake someone up during a light sleep, they will say, 'No, I wasn't asleep, I was busy thinking about something.'" REM sleep can often feel like you are awake, even if the person lying next to you swears you were dead to the world. From the inside it feels like thinking, from the outside it looks like sleeping. Evidently this phase of sleep can easily correspond with a type of consciousness.

The counterpart of this is NREM or non-REM sleep, during which there is no rapid eye movement. This phase is often called "deep sleep." All sorts of physical processes are put on the back burner; for instance, you breathe more gently and your heartrate is slower than during REM sleep.

On the sleep graph, this phase is characterized by long, regular loops: an EEG that looks completely different to one from an awake brain. These loops indicate that something special is going on in the brain, namely that many thousands of brain cells are changing electrical charge *at the same time*. In *Why We Sleep*, Matthew Walker uses a poetic image to illustrate it. Imagine a football stadium, he writes, full of thousands of fans. The people symbolize brain cells. They are usually speaking all at once, creating a chaotic cacophony. At some point that chatter fades away, and rhythmic chanting begins: the whole stadium is making the same noise at the same time and is quiet at the same time.

That's NREM sleep. Instead of carrying out all sorts of different activities side by side, a large number of brain cells are doing the same thing simultaneously. This coordinated activity is shown as large, slow waves on the sleep graph. This is very similar to what you see if someone is anesthetized or in a coma. Researchers who observed these waves on the EEG were therefore quick to draw the conclusion: when the waves are deep, there is no consciousness. That's why NREM is seen as deep, quiet sleep.

Another reason for NREM's reputation as your brain's ultimate state of rest is that if you wake up during this phase, you are much less likely to remember a dream than during REM sleep, and much more likely to say you were really asleep. That's where the distinction between dream sleep and deep sleep comes from.

REM and NREM are the most important phases of sleep, but that's by no means the whole picture. To start with, they alternate during every "sleep cycle": a block of sleep that consists of both REM and NREM sleep and lasts about ninety minutes. You have a number of these sleep cycles throughout the night, but they don't all have the same structure. At the beginning of the night, cycles consist of more deep sleep, for example, whereas towards the end they mainly consist of dream sleep.

Furthermore, REM and NREM are merely a rough way of dividing up the stages of sleep. Within NREM sleep alone, researchers differentiate between three, four, or even five sub-phases (NREM to NREM 5), which are increasingly deep. If you would like to read more about this, you will find a list of notes at the back of this book; I will stick to the most important distinction here, namely the difference between REM and NREM.[2]

They may appear to be opposites, but the contrast between dream sleep and deep sleep is less clear than it seems.

For example, it is quite possible to dream during deep sleep. If you understand dreaming to mean thinking of something while you sleep, you dream during *all* sleep phases and sub-phases.[3] Van Someren explains, "Even if you wake a good sleeper from their deepest sleep, two out of three times they will say: I was sleeping, but I was actually thinking about something. Sometimes that's all they can say, and other times they can tell you their whole chain of thoughts. Despite those slow waves on the EEG." Deep sleep waves may signify that someone is sleeping soundly, but that doesn't mean that their thoughts have stopped.

NREM's reputation as calm, unconscious sleep is therefore somewhat misleading. Not only do dreams take place during NREM, but it is also less serene than it seems. Bad nightmares, for example, only seem to happen in this deep phase of sleep: the deeper the sleep, the worse the nightmare. "Parasomnias"—striking behaviors such as sleepwalking, eating, talking, or even having sex in your sleep—also mainly occur in the deepest and last phase of NREM.[4]

The brainwaves of a patient in a coma or in vegetative sleep are also less peaceful than you might think, Van Someren explains. "Those brainwaves look very similar to sleep waves, and for years it was thought that there was no consciousness in either case. However, in 2005, a young woman who had ended up in a coma after a car accident, and was in a vegetative state, was put in an MRI scanner while researchers asked her to imagine playing tennis. Activity was detected in the cerebral cortex in the place responsible for planning physical activity.[5] Evidently she could hear them and respond to them through her brain activity—despite the fact she couldn't move and despite the fact there were slow brainwaves."

Since this case, great strides have been made with patients in the gray zone between life and death. Some of these patients appear to be conscious, even though you can't tell by looking at them. Brain scans show that they can carry out mental tasks, such as imagining themselves walking through each room in their house. Researchers can predict exactly where these thought exercises generate brain activity. If the patients respond in the same way as a healthy control group, this shows that they are responding to the task. In this way, it is possible to communicate with them. The researcher can ask, for example, "Are you in any pain? If the answer is no, imagine playing tennis." If the corresponding areas of the brain light up in the scan, the researcher knows that the patient is not in any pain.[6]

Sleep can feel like being awake, you can dream even in a deep sleep, and people who seem to be in an eternal vegetative state are not necessarily unconscious. In other words, sleep and consciousness are intricately intertwined and not mutually exclusive. In every phase, even in deep sleep, they overlap. And because sleep is so fluid, you can argue about whether or not someone is currently asleep.

Every now and then I stay over at a friend's house, who is at least as bad a sleeper as I am. At night, lying side by side in her large bed, we wish each other goodnight with the resignation of two colleagues with a long day of work ahead of us.

If I need to get up to go to the toilet, I try to slip out from under the duvet as carefully as possible and tiptoe across the wooden floor. She had been completely silent for a while, but now I hear her breathing a bit more deeply. I try my best not to wake her, but as soon as I raise a hand and the sheet rustles, her head shoots up from the pillow, as abruptly as a mousetrap slamming shut. "All right?" she asks. "Have you managed any sleep yet?" She hasn't. She's been lying awake mulling things over, she says; I try to reassure her that she was asleep.

I've only ever seen her catnap. During the day she is awfully attentive: she observes me as I break up my chocolate into tiny pieces, which I then eat one by one; she notices me hesitating for a quarter of a second before answering something and immediately asks what the matter is. Her attentiveness at night is equally uncanny. Her brain is a metropolis and there's always a light on somewhere.

I know how that feels from the inside too.

I remember one New Year's Eve, when we were staying in a converted hayloft somewhere in Catalonia. I had gone to lie down in the living room because I'd kept waking up whenever my boyfriend moved. But I couldn't sleep there either. I couldn't stop thinking about everything, planning every last detail of the garden of the house I didn't even own yet, wondering what to cook tomorrow, formulating a paragraph in my head. At some point I heard the floor creak; my boyfriend had come to see where I was. I could sense him standing beside the sofa and tried to say something, but to my surprise I was completely paralyzed. It was only when I was finally able to move and managed to emit a sleepy sound that I realized: I had been sleeping. I had been sleeping awake. And I could have sworn I hadn't slept a wink.

That kind of thing has happened to me on other occasions too. For example, when I was awake enough to hear the mosquito buzzing around my head, to feel it finally landing on my eyelid, but I was too asleep to shoo it away. It is a strange locked-in effect, whereby my mind is still switched on, but my body is disconnected from it. With a conscious effort, I can reconnect them. Am I asleep? It doesn't feel like it. Certainly not the next morning.

These are perhaps extreme examples, but sleep and consciousness are also more subtly intertwined. You might have fallen asleep in a noisy room, where fragments of the conversation around you were gradually incorporated into your dream. Or perhaps your bedroom has been filled with all sorts of strange goings-on and you only realized after a while that the talking dog telling you about a volcanic eruption was part of a dream, and that the sound of the eruption was caused by the bottle bank being emptied outside.

Sleep isn't a matter of either/or, a fact that can be observed in lots of animals, such as the birds that sleep with one eye and one half of their brain, while keeping a lookout for danger with the other eye. Fish in a school do something similar. They need sleep, like all animals, but still they keep on swimming, in perfect synchrony. How do they do it? What probably happens is that the fish on the edges of the school keep an eye on their surroundings so that the fish in the middle can navigate entirely through their spinal cords. They synchronize their movements with their neighbor's movements by reflex. Noticing whether a predatory fish is swimming nearby is another fish's job: these fish in the middle take a break and remain just awake enough in their sleep to be able to swim with the others.[7]

Humans too may find themselves carrying out their business half-asleep. Monotonous activities in particular are sometimes associated with brainwaves characteristic of light sleep. Soldiers on a long march, for example, may fall asleep but continue walking. A rhythmic activity can create a trance-like state, whereby you slip into sleep with your eyes open, without breaking your rhythm.

In addition, there is also something known as "microsleep." If you are very tired, part of your brain can switch off for just a moment. You are "gone" for a few seconds; your eyes close and your brain doesn't receive any information from your senses, meaning you don't see or hear anything. You don't usually realize you were temporarily asleep. However, a microsleep lasting two or three seconds can be dangerous— for example, if it happens while driving. Microsleep is the reason why a lack of sleep is responsible for one in five road traffic collisions.[8]

Conversely, the phenomenon of remaining alert while asleep is also observed in people, just like in other animals. If you study deep sleep (NREM) brainwaves, they appear less deep when people are sleeping in unfamiliar surroundings.

In these situations, one cerebral hemisphere stays a bit more awake than the other. That's why people often sleep restlessly in hotel rooms; they are latently aware that they are somewhere unfamiliar and that they ought to watch out.[9]

Researchers like Eus van Someren are interested in this type of latent awareness. "In addition to microsleep, where a part of your brain is 'switched off' for a moment, there is also something like micro-alertness," he says. This means that instead of your brain being asleep locally, there are wakeful parts here and there within a brain that is otherwise asleep. This could explain why so many insomniacs say they were awake, even though they appeared to be asleep to whoever was lying beside them—or on an EEG. Van Someren explains, "Perhaps a part of an insomniac's brain does remain active."

He uses the following simile to illustrate this process: "Sleep is like sailing in a submarine. What we see with insomniacs is that they keep surfacing for a very brief moment. They stick their submarine's periscope above water for a few seconds, as if to check that everything is all right."

So if anyone suggests you were just imagining those bad nights, remember that even sleep experts struggle to differentiate between being asleep and awake. There is a vast gray area between the two. It is hard to say where exactly in that area you might find yourself at night.

That's also why it's so difficult to fall asleep through willpower alone. Falling asleep is not like jumping off a diving board. You don't just take a step and suddenly find yourself underwater. Instead, insomniacs often get stuck somewhere between the two extremes of being wide awake and sleeping deeply.

And the main question, of course, is why?

09:00

HOURGLASS
AND CLOCK

WITH BAD SLEEPERS, the bodily processes that facilitate sleep may have gone awry. Your body naturally uses two instruments to make sure you sleep and to determine when this happens. You could think of them as the "clock" and the "hourglass."

The clock is your biological clock (which regulates your "circadian rhythm"). Thanks to that internal clock, all sorts of things in your body—such as your body temperature, level of alertness, appetite, and the production of hormones—follow a rhythm that is aligned with the planet's 24-hour cycle. Your biological clock ensures you are alert during the day and feel sleepy at night. If you have ever suffered from jet lag, you will know how it feels if this rhythm is compromised.

The second system your body uses to ensure you fall asleep at night is homeostasis. You could liken this to an hourglass. From the moment you wake up, your brain starts making adenosine, which accumulates over the hours that follow like sand in an hourglass. Your body uses this chemical to keep track of how long you have been up, and to increase the pressure to sleep accordingly. The more adenosine, the greater the urge to crawl into bed. That chemical is only broken down and the hourglass emptied when you fall asleep again.

If someone is having trouble sleeping, it seems logical to wonder whether there might be something wrong with their clock or hourglass. Eus van Someren spent years trying to find the answer to the question: What goes wrong with those two sleep regulation systems in the case of chronic insomniacs? "But actually, there wasn't anything to find," he says. "The few people who do have something wrong with their hourglass or biological clock often have sleep issues. But that's not the case for all insomniacs: the vast majority have well-functioning hourglasses and clocks, but still sleep badly."

There are other physical ailments that could keep you from your sleep, such as breathing issues (sleep apnea) or muscle spasms (restless legs syndrome), but these also only affect a small proportion of insomniacs, and don't explain the problems suffered by most of them.

Van Someren and his team therefore had to search elsewhere for the problem. They knew that insomnia is partly hereditary: if there are lots of bad sleepers in your direct family, you are significantly more likely to be one too. And they did indeed find a series of genes related to insomnia.

Which genes are they, and which processes do they control? The most logical way to find that out was to first compare them with genes already known to be associated with sleep. Perhaps there would be an overlap with the genes responsible for other aspects of sleep, such as whether you're an early bird or a night owl, how long you sleep for, if you enjoy taking naps, whether or not you snore... All of which are also inheritable.

But what Van Someren and his team discovered was surprising, he explains. "The overlap is negligible. The

genes related to insomnia have nothing to do with controlling sleep." In other words, regardless of where he
looked in the genes or physical processes that control
our sleep, he couldn't find anything anywhere to explain
chronic insomnia.

That is very interesting, because those physical processes
form the basis of most sleep tips. "Sleep hygiene" is all about
the habits that play havoc with your hourglass and clock;
drinking coffee tips over your hourglass, too much blue
light late in the day messes with your biological clock. However, with chronic insomniacs, these things don't seem to
be the real problem, and sleep hygiene therefore isn't the
real answer either.

Of course, if you are drinking ten cups of coffee a day and
it's taking you forever to get to sleep at night, cutting down
might help. However, as Van Someren also says, "Really bad
sleepers have typically been following all the tips for a long
time already, but to no avail."

We involuntary night owls are not simply too grubby for
Morpheus to share a bed with, so we don't need lecturing
about hygiene—or about valerian tablets, an even softer
pillow, or even thicker curtains. Our problem may not even
lie in *sleep* itself, but something else.

Van Someren expressed this even more strongly: "I am
becoming increasingly convinced that the whole idea that
insomnia is a *sleep* disorder was, in fact, an oversight."

My therapist already said I shouldn't focus on my sleep. It
was not only a waste of time, but it was also making my sleep
worse. Now I was hearing the same thing from the mouth
of a neuroscientist: sleep is not the problem.

That gave me a little shock, like when you are reading a thriller and suddenly realize that the suspect you had in mind couldn't have possibly done it. Now you have to start looking for another perpetrator. And just like in a good thriller, the answers were where I was least expecting them: not in the night, but in the day, hidden in plain sight.

10:00
HYPERAROUSAL

THERE IS CERTAINLY SOMETHING that sets involuntary night owls apart. If you subject an insomniac to a series of tests, you will notice that almost all of their measurable values are very high. Their brain is remarkably active. And that's not all; if you measure their heart rate, metabolic rate, or rate of breathing, or the level of stress hormones such as cortisol or adrenaline in their blood, or their body temperature, every single value will be high. If you ask them to fill in a questionnaire, they will report that they feel anxious and that they are very aware of what is going on both internally and in their environment. In other words, wherever you look, you find signs of a high level of alertness. That is the case at night, while they are lying awake, but—and this is important—it is also the case during the day. People with insomnia are *always* very alert, around the clock, whether they are awake or asleep.

This high level of alertness or arousal is called hyperarousal, and is a crucial factor in insomnia, Van Someren explains. At night, this high level of alertness comes down to the fact that the insomniac's brain is still too active for restful sleep. Above all, their dream sleep (REM sleep) is unstable; it is constantly interrupted. The periscope keeps on popping up above the water's surface.

Hyperarousal is also described as "an oversensitive stress system," my sleep therapist Sanne Verkooijen explains. Her PhD focused on the relationship between sleep problems and emotions, and she sees people like me in her practice on a daily basis.

Not everyone responds to an intense event in the same way, she says. "If you are confronted with a source of stress in your life, your stress system works more intensely than someone else's. You are more sensitive to it. I am sure you can imagine the effect that has on your sleep quality and why you are therefore much more susceptible to rumination, for example, than someone who responds less intensely."

This susceptibility can have all sorts of causes, she reveals. "It probably has a partially genetic basis, and could also be associated with the physical characteristics of your brain. A part of the brain called the orbitofrontal cortex is associated with alertness. It checks to see whether it's safe to sleep. If your orbitofrontal cortex makeup deviates a little from the norm, the feeling that it is okay to relax may not come as readily."

Furthermore, a sensitive stress system could be associated with your personality. "Some people like to be in control, for example, or have more neurotic tendencies than others, so they experience emotions and stimuli more intensely. A combination of these factors can make you prone to sleep problems."[1]

In *Why We Sleep*, Matthew Walker also claims that the insomniac's stress system (also called the sympathetic nervous system, which regulates the "fight-or-flight" response) is in overdrive, as a kind of physical malfunction.[2]

The stress system sets a whole series of physical reactions in motion: your heart rate increases, your brain becomes more active, your body temperature increases. All of these things make it more difficult to fall asleep. In order to initiate sleep, we need a lower body temperature, slower heart rate, less cortisol, and so on. It makes sense that the stress system counteracts these factors; after all, a stress response is *intended* to keep you alert and awake. If your stress response kicks in, your brain stays persistently alert and your senses stay "awake." And there you have it: insomnia.

I was once given a wake-up light (also known as a sunrise alarm), which comes on half an hour before your alarm and gradually brightens. It is designed to wake you up very slowly, but that's not how it worked with me. As soon as the light came on at the very lowest level, an almost imperceptible buzzing sound woke me up with a start. The whole point of a wake-up light is that you don't jolt awake, but that's exactly what I did. That's how vigilant I was in my sleep.

All too many times—crawling out of bed after yet another failed attempt to get some shut-eye—I have cursed myself for being "the way I am." A stress-head, too highly strung. And if you read the explanation above, as a bad sleeper, it's difficult not to become fatalistic. Genes, your personality, your brain: if insomnia is a result of that, you have a one-way ticket to exhaustion.

But there is a but—more about that in a moment. First of all, I want to make a brief aside to highlight the positive aspects of hyperarousal. Because even though it tears you up at night, this ultra-alertness has benefits during the day.

11:00

THE BRIGHT SIDE
OF HYPERAROUSAL

IF YOU LOOK at the research into sleep deprivation, it doesn't seem possible that someone can sleep terribly night after night and still function. I got the same impression from Els van der Helm, who told me how bad interrupted nights are for your ability to think logically, learn things, and maintain self-restraint. If I put these findings and my own sleeping pattern side by side, I can conclude that by now I should be walking into walls like a fool, with the memory of a goldfish. But I function, just like the majority of insomniacs. How is that possible?

Van Someren sheds light on this too. "What you need to know about research into the effects of a lack of sleep is that this kind of research is almost always carried out on people who, in principle, sleep well," he says. They are often student volunteers, for example, who make easy test subjects for their professors. These students are then kept up for a number of hours each night for the duration of the study, before being subjected to tests. "It is much less common that a specially selected group of insomniacs is used for this kind of research. However, the *conclusions* are often extended to people suffering from insomnia. They don't get enough sleep either, right? What usually happens is that the two groups are lumped together: people who can sleep well, but simply aren't getting enough sleep, and 'real' insomniacs."[1]

That is actually a very peculiar thing to do, because these two groups respond completely differently to a lack of sleep. Good sleepers who are kept awake for a number of nights certainly perform disastrously at all sorts of tests. However, if the insomniacs perform the same tests, the results are completely different.

"If, as an exception, you carry out a study like this on insomniacs, what you find is that they don't perform disastrously at all. If you try really hard, you can find a *couple* of areas where it has been found that insomniacs perform *slightly* worse than others. However, it is fascinating just how well they do. They are faster and perform better at certain cognitive tasks than people without insomnia. Despite sleeping badly for nights on end."

Not well rested, but alert nonetheless. In order to see how that is possible, Van Someren did the opposite of a sleep deprivation study, by getting bad sleepers to sleep *better* as opposed to keeping them up. "First of all, we spent two months intensively treating bad sleepers. We used cognitive behavioral therapy, bright light in the morning, more exercise ... A military sleep regimen, which helped them sleep *a bit* better. When we got them to perform cognitive tasks after this regimen, they performed better than before, and significantly better than the healthy control group without any sleep problems," Van Someren explains.[2]

His hypothesis: "People with sleep problems have a brain that is very well-trained in paying attention. This could be due to all sorts of factors: a genetic predisposition, experiences in their early childhood, or perhaps it is associated with certain features of their brain stem, or the amount of a specific signalling chemical in the brain: noradrenaline. We don't know exactly. In any case, for whatever reason, these people have constructed mental motorways for vigilance, as opposed to country roads.

"If your brain is that alert, it becomes very difficult to switch off that system. You don't suddenly get a different brain the moment you crawl into bed. So there you lie, with your motorways for paying attention, and you notice every sound and every heartbeat."

What may be a handicap at night is often an advantage during the day. These mental motorways, Van Someren explains, are useful when it comes to things such as attentiveness, learning, and problem-solving. It is childish, but it gave me a boost to think of insomnia like that: the dark underside of a medal that shines extra brightly during the day.

Of course, I wasn't the first to take comfort in that idea. In fact, among my colleagues—writers, who have made their livelihoods through attentiveness—insomnia is often seen as something inseparable from their work.

My favorite reason to lie awake is because something in my mind is coming to life. For example, during the feverish weeks in which I "discover" a new idea for a novel. Or when, after toiling away for ages, I suddenly work out the book's structure and know exactly how it's going to end. All sorts of things suddenly seem to come together; the text I am working on is linked to everything I see, read, think, or remember. Anything can serve as inspiration, nothing can pass me by: I am acutely focused all day long. There is suddenly a reality behind the reality, of which I get glimpses and whose coherence and meaning I try to translate onto paper. Intact, without squeezing the life out of it, because it keeps moving. Like trying to move a spider's web without evicting the spider.

And that keeps me awake. Or actually more than awake: incandescent. Doubly awake, for myself and my fictional company. That alertness seems to be the price I pay for a good text.

If it didn't lead to such fatigue, I would work every night in that strange vacuum in which no one disturbs you. Overnight hours are hours that don't actually exist, because no one else takes part in them. It is as if they are outside time, they are only for you, jokers to play as you choose. Writing in the night is reckless. Almost every text I have written that a reader has ever called "bold" came about at night.

Even the despair that goes hand in hand with insomnia is a weapon: in the decided illogicality of the night, it seems like nothing can happen that's worse than what's already happening. You are awake, you can't sleep, you feel like you're slowly going mad. So who cares?

In contrast to this are the weeks or months in which I try in vain to develop a project. The text stalls as soon as it appears on paper and I can no longer get it moving again. Then too I am acutely focused and that also keeps me up at night, but without any pleasure.

Without reading a word, my boyfriend knows if what I am writing is any good. He can tell from how I am, how I act. He can tell from how I sleep, and the way in which I lie awake. If it is "alive" he notices that; and if it's a nonstarter, he feels me kicking around in the overheated bed.

For me, writing is an attempt to assign meaning to what I experience and what I see of the world. As a poor sleeper, it's my good fortune that writing sometimes means my insomnia is meaningful too.

As mentioned earlier, I am not the first writer to take comfort in my nocturnal output, and maybe even get a sense of superiority from it. Nabokov, who wore his insomnia as a badge of honor, is the classic example. In his autobiography, he ridicules the "people on trains, who lay their newspaper aside, fold their silly arms, and immediately, with an offensive familiarity of demeanour, start snoring." He describes sleep itself as a "nightly betrayal of reason, humanity, genius."[3]

Nabokov is quite something, but I don't know anyone who goes further in their praise of insomnia than the Romanian-French philosopher Emil Cioran, who became known for his dismal world view. He spoke in interviews about his first, intense period of insomnia, which started when he was about twenty. He didn't sleep for weeks on end and instead wandered the streets of Bucharest. It was during those nights, he said, that all sorts of ideas came to him, for which he later found fame.

He was plagued with insomnia his entire life, even if "plagued" isn't quite the right word to describe Cioran's intense hatred *and* love of his insomnia. On one hand, it almost drove him to suicide on several occasions. He described the pain and exhaustion that followed; how every sound became a shout, every touch a stab. The night exaggerates every misery and Cioran did so too: What was a single crucifixion compared with the daily crucifixion of the insomniac? What was such pain compared with nights like his, which even the most ingenious torturer couldn't have thought up?

But he also saw insomnia as the greatest experience of his life, as his personal revelation, and even as the only source of true knowledge. He believed that insomnia made the mind exceptionally sharp. Cioran wasn't familiar with the term hyperarousal and he would have probably found it too ordinary anyway, but his praise of insomnia certainly brings it to mind. As he wrote in *On the Heights of Despair*, a book he penned in French, the key feature of his sleepless nights was a *lucidité vertigineuse*—a dizzying lucidity.[4] Insomnia sheds light on truths from which sleep would otherwise protect you. It provides an insight you don't want to have at all, but which you keep seeking in spite of yourself.

As a result of this clarity, you ought to assess thinkers according to their number of sleepless nights, he claimed. The more sleepless, the clearer the mind and the more valuable the thinker. In this way he also elevated his own insomnia, which he often emphasized and which he wrote about for his entire life, to a sign of his exceptionality.

Incidentally, he was well aware of his own Stockholm syndrome. If you don't sleep for long enough, Cioran said, "You don't feel like a human being similar to others, as others live in a state of unconsciousness. So then, you start developing a tremendous ego. You say to yourself, 'My destiny is different, I now have the experience of uninterrupted wakefulness.' Only that pride, the pride of a catastrophe, gives you courage then. You cultivate the extraordinary feeling that you are no longer part of ordinary humanity."[5]

If human beings are the only animal that lies awake, Cioran believed, insomnia is the characteristic that defines humanity. The more insomniac, the more human.[6]

I think I understand how he came to that idea: there is something enchanting about the sense of intensified presence that insomnia can give you. If you are sufficiently tired, you reach the limits of your wakefulness. Your consciousness has been spread out over too many hours like butter over too much toast. It becomes impossible to carry on as usual.

At precisely that point it sometimes seems as if you are breaking through something, and only then do you truly wake up. Instead of losing consciousness, you transition to the other extreme: supra-alertness, an almost unbearable sensitivity. It seems as if you hear more, see more, feel more, think more, and understand more than ever. It is the insomniac's consolation prize.

There are probably few insomniacs to whom their condition is as special and valuable as insomniac authors.[7] But even if you do away with the poetic exaggeration, they all refer to the bright side shared by others with hyperarousal, which I didn't want to leave unmentioned.

But for those gritting their teeth as they toss and turn, I shall return to the matter of understanding sleep. How does hyperarousal come about, and can you restrain that roving mind?

12:00
UNPROCESSED
EMOTIONS

THERE IS SOMETHING STRANGE about using hyperarousal to explain insomnia. Very well, you are extremely alert, and you can't sleep as a result. But is that not the same as saying that the air is moving very quickly, and that it is windy as a result? It is circular reasoning, which in itself fails to provide an explanation. Where does this restlessness *come from*?

If you try to answer this question by looking at the brain, two factors are very important: the signalling chemical noradrenaline, and how this chemical influences emotional processing. This processing often goes awry with insomniacs, Eus van Someren explains.

One of the things that sleep usually does is "tidy up" the day's emotions for you. They are literally, physically, assigned to another place in your brain, after which you experience them less intensely. Your dream sleep, or REM sleep, is especially good at that.

"Sleep is good at reorganizing connections in your brain," Van Someren explains. "At night, the previous day's experiences are processed and assigned to a different place in your brain. Sometimes, connections between brain cells need to be broken for this. There is one state in which the brain has a very special opportunity to do that, and that's REM sleep."

That phase of sleep is unique because it is the only time a particular chemical is not present in the brain: noradrenaline. I mentioned it earlier. Noradrenaline reinforces the connections between brain cells; you can think of it as a kind of glue that sticks the connections firmly together. It is a signalling chemical that is also associated with stress.

If noradrenaline is absent, connections between brain cells can be easily removed and reorganized. That is what happens during REM sleep; because noradrenaline is not being produced in the brain, existing connections can be broken and there's a chance for information to pass through the brain through other routes. Intense experiences, for example, also get their "place": they are processed and stored somewhere else, and are therefore no longer in the forefront of your mind.

Each experience you have triggers a reaction in your brain by activating your brain's emotional circuit. Imagine, for example, that someone shows you a video of you singing really badly; the embarrassment you feel when you watch it can be seen as activity on a brain scan. When, after some sleep, you think about that experience or see the same clip again, the emotional circuit won't kick in to the same extent as the first time. It is as if the emotion has been washed out of the memory during the night.[1]

However, this whole process can also go wrong. Van Someren explains, "What we think is going on with insomniacs is that there is a problem with their noradrenaline. The nucleus in the brain that produces noradrenaline—the locus coeruleus—may remain slightly active even during REM sleep." This means that noradrenaline keeps flowing through the brain during this phase too. As a result, the brain stays alert. Hence the hyperarousal and hence the periscope that keeps popping up above the surface. However, that's not all.

The presence of noradrenaline makes it very difficult to cut off and reclassify connections between brain cells. This means that the "tidying up" of emotions doesn't work because everything remains stuck. Try tidying something up with glue on your fingers. "It is possible that with insomniacs, the connections that would usually be separated are actually further strengthened because of this noradrenaline. Instead of disposing of emotions, the brain keeps hold of them even more intensely. And that means that your emotional brain— BAM!—flares up whenever you remember certain things."[2] You feel a lot, and you *keep* feeling a lot. That keeps you up.[3]

It is not only the case that sleeping doesn't help get rid of those feelings; the restless sleep you get as an insomniac could even be making things worse. The fragmentary REM sleep that broken sleepers get doesn't seem to help tidy up stress or other emotions. Instead, it does precisely the opposite, Van Someren explains. "The more restless REM sleep they have had, the more intensely their emotional brain is activated the next day."[4] The details are not yet completely clear. But there is something in their brain, or rather in their dream sleep, which is obstinately holding on to those emotions. The feelings are left lying around, and the insomniac trips over them on their way to sleep.

13:00
INSOMNIA, ANXIETY, AND DEPRESSION

IT IS NOT JUST INSOMNIACS who are affected by noradrenaline and restless REM sleep. The same applies to people suffering from depression, anxiety disorders, or trauma. These conditions are also associated with REM sleep that is different from usual: it is unstable and constantly interrupted. As a result, emotions are not processed normally.

Van Someren mentioned this as a side note, but when I probed him, he explained that there is a huge overlap between the pathologies of insomnia, depression, and anxiety disorder. "If you look at all the complaints that go hand in hand with these conditions, which is what epidemiological studies do, the overlap seems to be about 80 percent." It can be seen as one big cluster of symptoms, as opposed to three separate conditions. A big, restless, dark malaise that you can give different names to. "What I suspect," he says, "is that with anxiety, depression, and insomnia, the same thing is going on in the brain: REM sleep is working counterproductively. Emotions are therefore not being processed and start to accumulate instead. Perhaps only small differences determine *which* emotion is retained. Some people will mainly suffer from persistent anxiety, others from a sense of hopelessness, and others still will notice they mainly carry stress over to the following day." Which emotion is retained determines whether someone is more likely to recognize themselves in the diagnosis of an anxiety disorder, depression, or a sleeping disorder.

The fact that insomnia, depression, and anxiety manifest themselves in such similar ways during sleep obviously caught my attention. I mentioned earlier that I was able to choose which diagnosis I wanted; according to the psychologist, my sleeping disorder could just as easily have been an anxiety disorder. The symptoms were obviously similar enough. Now I was learning that both disorders also manifest in the brain in similar ways—a family resemblance they also share with depression. And that's a diagnosis I'd *also* had before, when I first went to the doctor with sleeping problems about ten years ago.

As a result, my quest for sleep was inadvertently broadened. In addition to insomnia, anxiety and depression had now also suddenly become part of my attempts to understand sleep.

I soon learned that these three disorders are not only characterized by similar complaints; they are similar in other ways too.

We already saw that genes that make you susceptible to insomnia are not related to other inheritable characteristics of your sleep. At the time, this seemed like a disappointing result of Van Someren's research, but this genetic dead-end led him down another avenue. "The genes that make someone susceptible to insomnia are not related to sleep. But they are very similar to the genes that make someone susceptible to mood disorders, such as anxiety or depression, or to the characteristics associated with these disorders, such as neuroticism."[1]

It is not a coincidence that the archetypal insomniac is a melancholic.[2] This old stereotype is also seen in modern science's figures and tables, since depressive people also tend to suffer from sleep problems. Three quarters of them have insomnia, while others sleep too much (hypersomnia), and their sleep is structured differently from usual. Disturbed sleep is such an important characteristic that some researchers believe that depression should not be diagnosed if sleep complaints are not present.[3]

However, that is not all. Insomnia is a powerful predictor of suicide,[4] and sleep problems are characteristic of almost all mental disorders. The overlap is so great that they seem to originate from the same source. There is virtually no pathology in which someone is feeling down, anxious, confused, or has other mental struggles, but is still sleeping really well.

It won't come as a surprise to most people that there is such a strong link between sleep and mood. You are probably familiar with it from your own experience, even if it's simply a case of feeling a bit grumpy after a bad night's sleep. The most striking thing about the large overlap to which Van Someren refers is that science goes to such trouble to strictly separate the gloomy triad of anxiety, depression, and insomnia. They must be separated per se—even if these complaints are present in the same person. The idea behind this is that if you can study each complaint in isolation, the results of your research will be purer.[5]

For research into insomnia, for example, anyone who has depressive complaints as well as sleeping problems is usually removed from the test group, despite the fact that these complaints almost always go hand in hand. "That's how we did it ten years ago at the Dutch Brain Institute," Van Someren says. "We were looking for insomniacs for a study; we found 470 and got them to fill in questionnaires to determine how anxious or depressed they were. We then removed anyone who was also a bit anxious or depressed, with the lowest possible threshold value for those pathologies, even if those people all really had insomnia too. Ultimately we were left with 35 people: the Vikings among the insomniacs. Well, we did some great studies with those people, but the results don't say much at all about *all* insomniacs."

Someone like me would have been removed from the study, so do the results actually apply to me?

That's the question, Van Someren says. This type of exclusion means sleep researchers struggle to establish whether one group of insomniacs can be used as the basis for drawing conclusions about sleep for a different group. His team therefore turned the reasoning around. "Instead of strictly selecting people who only had sleep complaints, we considered *everyone* who slept badly." They opened an online "sleep register," where hundreds of thousands of night owls signed themselves up for a study. All of those people filled in a large number of questionnaires, which weren't just about sleep. "Each and every characteristic that had ever been associated with insomnia was included."

Since casting their net as widely as possible, Van Someren and his research team have made great strides.[6] "It was a huge blind spot. Anxiety researchers had been looking at the day, sleep researchers the night. Even if they were often studying the same person."

14:00
SLEEP
AND MOOD

I AM FAMILIAR with the interconnectedness of sleeping problems and low mood. In periods of intense insomnia, much of what I see and think is bleak. It is as if all of that staring into the surrounding darkness rubs off on me, so everything appears gloomy, day and night.

Nowadays, we want to explain this kind of thing by referring to the brain. We can do so in various ways. In the previous chapter, Eus van Someren suggested that noradrenaline interferes with REM sleep, and in doing so also affects the way in which emotions are processed. Sleep and mood complaints therefore originate from the same "error" in the brain.[1]

However, there are also other ways neuroscientists explain the large overlap between sleep problems and depression. A popular hypothesis, for example, is that mood disorders are a result of sleep deprivation; your brain responds badly to a lack of sleep, which over time causes your emotions to go haywire.

Peter Meerlo explains how exactly that could work. He is a neurobiologist at the University of Groningen, and carries out research into sleep and mood disorders. He animatedly confirms that there is a strong link between sleep deprivation and low mood.

"Long-running studies show that people with sleep problems are two to four times more likely to become depressed than your average person," Meerlo explains.[2] "We therefore believe that disturbed sleep can upset your mood." This has been the prevailing thought in research into the link between mood and sleep for decades.

What is the reasoning behind this? Sleep is probably necessary in order for the brain to repair itself (for example to clear up waste products and to maintain connections between neurons). If your brain doesn't get the chance to do this, it slowly develops problems. Experiments on animals suggest that at least three things go wrong in terms of mood and emotions in the event of sleep deprivation: the brain becomes less sensitive to the signalling chemical serotonin, the hippocampus shrinks, and the amygdala runs riot.

First: serotonin. This is a neurotransmitter: a chemical that transfers signals in the brain. You can think of it as an envelope containing information, which is delivered and read by other brain cells. "Serotonin is an important signalling chemical that is involved in almost every process in your brain, including controlling your mood," Meerlo explains. If someone's mood is messed up, there may be something wrong with their serotonin system. The postman is lazy, the letterboxes are congested, lots of post is getting lost. That's called emotional dysregulation. Something like that may be what's going on in people with depression.

And what about people who aren't getting enough sleep? Meerlo explains, "My research so far has looked at the sensitivity of serotonin receptors in rats. The human brain is the next step. We know that if you keep rats awake for long enough, their receptors gradually become less sensitive to serotonin, which is exactly what we see with depressive patients." Insofar as serotonin is concerned, the sleep-deprived brain of a rat is therefore similar to the depressive brain.

The second part of the brain that runs into issues in the event of sleep deprivation is the hippocampus. "That seahorse-shaped part of the brain is one of the few parts of an adult brain that still regularly produces new cells," Meerlo explains. In all likelihood, these new cells help the hippocampus carry out its most important tasks: learning and memory formation. However, this part of the brain is also involved in emotions, as memory and emotions are connected. "That's why you remember intensely felt things more clearly. In other words, the most important traces of memory we form are linked to emotions. It follows that the hippocampus communicates very emphatically with parts of the brain where emotions are generated and processed," Meerlo says. "If the hippocampus is impaired, you run into issues with the regulation of emotions and the formation of emotional memories." Apart from memory problems, a malfunctioning hippocampus therefore also generates symptoms of low mood.

The sleep-deprived brain looks similar to the depressive brain in this regard too. In people with depression, the hippocampus often doesn't function as effectively and is smaller, as if it has shrunk—and it is possible that the same also applies to people who aren't getting enough sleep. Meerlo says, "Just like with serotonin, we asked: Can disturbed sleep lead to a smaller hippocampus? If you chronically disturb the sleep of laboratory animals, you do see that their hippocampus shrinks."

A third important emotional center in the brain that suffers from a lack of sleep is the amygdala, an almond-shaped part of the brain that helps coordinate your emotional responses. Even after a single night of sleep deprivation, the amygdala appears to become overactive. "You will be familiar with that—that you become a bit uninhibited after a bad night's sleep," Meerlo says. You speak before you think, or burst into tears. That could be due to the fact that the amygdala is no longer under control.[3]

In summary, laboratory animals that are kept awake for long periods of time face a three-stage rocket launch of gradual changes in the brain: fewer sensitive serotonin receptors, a shrunken hippocampus, and an overactive amygdala. All of these changes are also seen in people with depression.

I want to make three side notes here. First of all, it is assumed that it is the sleep deprivation that causes the rats to suffer, as opposed to the stress of the chronic harassment used to keep them awake.[4]

Second, it remains to be seen whether the findings from these experiments on laboratory animals can also be applied to humans. And third, whether the effects would be the same for "good" sleepers who are kept awake as for insomniacs—the difference Van Someren referred to earlier.

As mentioned, the theory that depression is a result of disturbed sleep has been dominant for decades. However, other researchers argue that it is precisely the other way round: sleep complaints are not a cause, but a symptom of depression. In all likelihood, the relationship between sleep problems and depression works both ways: one can reinforce the other in a vicious circle in which cause and effect cannot be separated.[5]

And there is a third option too: they both originate from the same unknown source, whereby sleep problems are often the first complaint, announcing the coming depression like a rising wind announces the storm.[6]

I could have stopped at the neurological explanations I have outlined here. I could have thought: it's probably my amygdala or my hippocampus; or it's my overactive stress system that's making me feel anxious and stressed out; or it's my noradrenaline, and the fragmented REM sleep associated with it, which is causing so many emotions to hang around.[7] In other words: it's my brain. How unfortunate. An error I can't do anything about.

If you view insomnia as a neurologist does, you can arrive at a nice, clear explanation: something is going wrong in your brain, causing you to sleep badly and triggering emotions that prevent your daily life from running smoothly.

However, I am not satisfied with a neurological explanation. Perhaps that is the professional bias of the writer; if I include a character in a book, I don't explain their behavior and emotions on the basis of signalling chemicals or brain defects. Nor do I do so for the behavior of enemies and friends. Perhaps my dissatisfaction is simply due to the human need for meaning. For me, neurological explanations do not provide the whole picture. The most important question they leave unanswered is that of the *content* of those disruptive emotions. As such, they deny the possibility that there is a reason for those emotions: that they are useful.

Eus van Someren's research team speaks of a failed "neutralization" of emotions.[8] As if we are talking about unpleasant smells that you need to conceal with air freshener.

However, I am accustomed to thinking that emotions are relevant reactions to whatever is going on in my life or around me, and that I need to do something with them if I smell disaster. This need provokes the questions: Where do these emotions come from? Are they justifiable? And is it perhaps even possible that the mind has a *reason* why it isn't letting go of these emotions, but instead stubbornly keeping them in the foreground?

Pain is generally seen as something useful. If you feel your fingers burning, you quickly withdraw your hand and prevent worse injury. Psychological pain can work in exactly the same way. However, as soon as you label it a "disorder," it becomes much more difficult to find anything positive or useful about it.[9]

Insomnia as
an Alarm

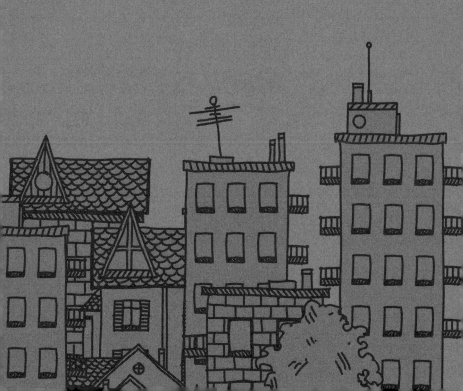

15:00
INSOMNIA ISN'T SIMPLY A DEFECT

MATTHEW WALKER uses an interesting description to explain insomnia: an overactive stress system.

Overactive. As if insomniacs are houses with overly sensitive alarms that go off every time a cat walks past. Overactive implies something that is exceptional, unusual, or abnormal. By doing so, Walker articulates a commonplace idea in today's narrowly scientific view of sleep that you see time and again on popular websites and in the media: there is something wrong with insomniacs. Either their sleep hygiene is lacking, or their brains are acting abnormally. For the insomniac, this translates as: either you are doing something wrong, or there is something wrong with you. The world around you has nothing to do with it.

Thus, insomnia is invariably reduced to a *biological* matter, a problem with the individual body and brain.

An advantage to telling insomniacs their problem is physical is that the approach for dealing with it is relatively straightforward: practical tips for sleeping, better sleep hygiene, or medication. You have a physical oversensitivity; your body is producing too many stress responses. You were unlucky; there was an error in your design: here's a pill or a list of practical tips. Dim your smartphone and buy new curtains. Apart from that, nothing major has to change, and the pharmaceutical companies and other sellers of sleep can make a good sum of money out of you. Great solution.

Only that isn't a solution. Those new curtains don't help you, the tablets don't have much effect. So you end up with a chemical hangover, convinced you are condemned to sleeping badly forevermore because of your genes, brain, or personality. This belief is a dead end, a life sentence.

Fortunately, there are arguments for seeing things differently. The first is the huge *number* of chronic insomniacs.

Imagine a motorway. Somewhere, in the middle of a vast plateau of meadows, the road bends. Cars are constantly racing past. However, something strange is going on: out of every nine cars that go around the bend, one spins off the road. Every ninth car is done for. The crumpled metal piles up at the side of the motorway.

A group of experts is sent to the scene to find out what's going on. They take cutting-edge equipment with them, subject the car wrecks to numerous investigations, and debate the cause of the chaos. Ultimately, they produce a well-argued report. Their conclusion: there is something wrong with one in nine cars.

That's more or less how many sleep experts diagnose bad sleepers. Walker—Mr. Overactive Stress System—writes that approximately one in nine meet the strict clinical definition of insomnia.[1]

One in nine.[2]

When I read that, I was struck by how high the figure was. Too high for it to be something exceptional. Could one in nine people really have an unusual, "broken" stress system? Could a function like sleep, so crucial to health and functioning, be that badly affected by bad luck with genes and brain design for one in nine individuals of a species?[3]

That is possible. But for a problem that is so systemic, it seems logical to me to also look at the system in which that brain exists: the society, the context, whatever you want to call it. The road, in which there may be a peculiar bend.

Another thing that is striking about sleep problems is that they are not evenly distributed throughout the population, the same way car accidents are not evenly distributed along a route. In France, highway fatalities are marked by haunting man-sized figures at the side of the road. It's as if those shadowy men seek each other out; here and there you find a gloomy congregation on the roadside.

That type of congregation is also characteristic of insomniacs. It is striking how the approximately ten percent of insomniacs among us are not evenly distributed along the axes of gender, ethnicity, or professional situation.

On average, women have more sleeping problems than men[4]—a difference that becomes apparent at puberty and for which no neurological or genetic explanation has yet been found. Ethnicity also appears to play a role when it comes to sleep. Dutch people with an immigrant background are more likely to have sleep problems.[5] In the United States, people from Latin American or Black communities are also significantly more likely to have sleep problems than their white fellow citizens,[6] and to get less sleep.[7] (More about this in chapters 20:00 and 23:00.)

Finally, it has been established that how you make your living is also important. There are big differences in terms of sleep between employed and unemployed people. I will return to this later.

It is unlikely that "errors" in the brain or stress system would be distributed so unevenly throughout the population, especially because they often affect groups in our society with greater socioeconomic difficulties.

Another argument for not obsessing about the brain is the fact that sleep problems are on the rise. Not only are they very prevalent; they are evidently occurring *more often* too.

Statistics Netherlands recently reported that the number of Dutch people with sleep problems rose by 3 percent in one year—from 21 percent in 2017 to 24 percent in 2018.[8] It is not yet clear whether this trend is continuing; not enough large-scale research has been carried out into this in the Netherlands as yet. Figures from other countries over the past decades certainly suggest that this is the case.[9] The Brits report almost twice as many insomnia diagnoses in 2007 as 1993[10] and the Norwegians saw the percentage of their population with insomnia increase by 30 percent between 2000 and 2010.[11] The Chinese saw their average night shortened by 1.5 hours over the last decade.[12] Sleep complaints and insomnia increased by 8 percent among American adults between 2002 and 2012, and by 30 to 50 percent among young adults during the same decade.[13] Researchers note an increasing trend towards short sleep since then.[14] These findings aren't uncontroversial, as there is also research suggesting there has only been a small decrease in American sleep, or none at all.[15] Since the pandemic, the average American may even be spending slightly *more* time in bed, although not necessarily sleeping better.[16] However, data from the National Health Interview Surveys show a decrease in sleep duration over the years, especially among Black people and Mexican Americans.[17] Sleep isn't getting any easier, if sales of sleeping aids are anything to go by; sales of melatonin—a hormonal supplement supposed to help you fall asleep—more than doubled in the U.S. between 2017 and 2020.[18] Internationally, 44 percent of adults say they feel their sleep has worsened in recent years.[19]

The expression "sleeping like a child" also seems to risk acquiring new meaning, since children and teenagers especially seem to be having increasing trouble. The U.K. has recently seen a sharp rise in hospital admissions for children with sleep disorders, with a near doubling of cases over seven years.[20] Sleep problems are on the rise among young teenagers in Finland, Iceland, Denmark, and Sweden.[21] Dutch sleep clinics indicate that they are seeing increasing numbers of primary and secondary school children with serious complaints; this increase has even been described as "explosive."[22] Figures from Amsterdam, where sleep problems are twice the usual Dutch rate, reveal that young people in cities are sleeping particularly badly: of Amsterdam's Millennials, four in ten have problems with their sleep. Only two in ten young adults in Amsterdam are *satisfied* with their sleep.[23]

Incidentally, it is not just sleep that is suffering: the World Health Organization notes a worldwide increase in anxiety disorders and depression too.[24]

The fact that sleeping problems appear to be getting bigger is difficult to reconcile with the purely neurological explanation of "an error in your brain." Would we spontaneously develop more brain errors en masse? Has our sleep hygiene really become that poor? Or does our changing world have a part to play?[25]

Because yes, the world is changing. And in 2020 it changed spectacularly, a radical reordering that shows little sign of abating several years later. While the pandemic transformed our daily lives, it also changed our nights: we collectively started lying awake more.

In Google Trends, you can investigate how often a particular search term has recently been entered. For example, interest in the term "insomnia" peaks nightly at 3:00 AM, but zooming out, you see larger trends. If I type in *insomnia*, for example, looking at a multiple-year period, the jagged line shoots up around mid-March 2020. That's when many countries went into lockdown. Interest in the search term "insomnia" soared internationally in the early months of the pandemic, and increased in tandem with the cumulative number of COVID-related deaths.[26]

At around the same time, I saw articles pop up here and there about *coronavirus insomnia*. Express Scripts, a major American pharmacy organization, reported a sharp increase in the use of sedatives and tranquilizers between mid-February and mid-March 2020, with a peak in the week in which the World Health Organization declared the beginning of the pandemic. The use of anti-anxiety medications and antidepressants increased dramatically too, by 34 and 19 percent respectively.[27] In Canada, sleep problems rose from 36 percent before the pandemic to more than 50 percent.[28] We are only beginning to understand the impact this pandemic will have on sleep in the long run.[29]

A trend like that cannot be explained by the neurological account of insomnia due to genetic susceptibility, or from an excess of certain signalling chemicals in the brain—unless that type of excess can come about as a response to the news.[30]

Of course, that context plays a role. You always lie down *somewhere* to sleep. You always lie awake worrying about *something*.

Furthermore, emotions are known to play a major role in sleeping problems. Who hasn't lain awake at night thinking about an argument, work stress, money worries, or a broken heart? If you are going through a hard time emotionally, you'll have more trouble sleeping, and serious sleeping problems are sometimes the result.[31] There is good reason why the two most common triggers of insomnia are *worry* and *anxiety*.[32]

If that is the case, why is there such a focus on physical, neurological causes? The strange thing is that lots of sleep experts acknowledge that psychological problems are a key cause of bad sleep, but they draw an illogical conclusion from that fact. Matthew Walker writes (I have added the italics): "Since *psychological* distress is a principal instigator of insomnia, researchers have focused on examining the *biological* causes that underlie emotional turmoil." He is referring here to the physical characteristics of the brain and the rest of the nervous system.[33]

I had to read that sentence three times, as it is a very peculiar way of thinking. *Emotions* are key, so we go and look at *physical* characteristics?

How about going and looking at those emotions? After all, a considerable number of us evidently have such turbulent emotions that we are unable to sleep.

Taking all these considerations into account, I became convinced that I had to look at my insomnia in a different way. Did the times in which I struggled most not coincide with heartbreak, financial concerns, or other turbulence? However, if I am honest, something else also played a role: frustration. I couldn't come to terms with the idea that my insomnia was not only pointless, but also irreversible.

What if my brain isn't malfunctioning, but is instead responding meaningfully to my situation? What if the alertness characteristic of the insomniac is not *caused* by changes in the brain, but *reflected* in those changes? What if the overlap between sleeping problems and mood problems means that there are things that make us sad *and* keep us awake at the same time? If that's the case, insomnia might not be a meaningless defect, but a meaningful signal. An error message that isn't indicating something is wrong with the brain, but with the world in which that brain exists.[34]

Perhaps insomniacs aren't oddballs, but oracles.

16:00
SLEEP IN
THE SPOTLIGHT

IN THE EIGHTEENTH CENTURY, as artificial lighting advanced and Europe's major cities installed tens of thousands of gas lamps to light their streets, people put darkness behind themselves symbolically too. Mysticism and superstition became a thing of the past; from then, reason ruled.

Reason, or rationality, was redefined; it relied on facts and observations. The emphasis on what was visible and controllable had major consequences on what could be considered "science," and what it focused on. Only those things that could be precisely measured were still rational.

This view, which still prevails today, has proved very beneficial to us, resulting in huge progress in the fields of medicine and technology, for example. However, it also makes us blind to certain things. After all, this rational perspective dictates that everything should be approached in a natural scientific manner, including the fields that perhaps don't lend themselves to this, such as the study of the human psyche. When considering feelings and emotions in psychology or psychiatry, all research results must be generalizable and based on objective and value-free research and exact measurements. Even when dealing with something like sleeping problems, the objective remains to find universal laws that always apply—just think of gravity.

However, that's illogical, if not impossible. At least that's what psychoanalyst Darian Leader believes. Leader is a slender, bespectacled Brit whose book *Why Can't We Sleep?* makes a fiery response to Matthew Walker's *Why We Sleep*.

Leader argues that the attempt to explain insomnia through natural scientific methods impoverishes our view of it. The empirical approach means that medical attention focuses exclusively on the body, particularly the brain. After all, the body is visible and tangible; you can cut it open, measure it, and understand it. It is much more difficult to carry out scientific research into something intangible like the human mind. No one has ever seen a spirit, so what's an enlightened scientist to do?

The reflexive reaction, even in psychiatry, is therefore to assume that the cause is physical, even when dealing with mental complaints.[1] Neurons and genes can, at least, be measured. But emphasizing measurability creates a blind spot; causes that may *not* be in the body and brain, such as personal experiences or social context, tend to be disregarded. It is difficult to isolate them and complex to measure and compare them effectively.[2] Just think of your own situation: it is so multifaceted that you wouldn't have enough space to describe it in a hefty novel and there's no way you could generalize and compare it in a natural scientific manner with another insomniac's situation. The customary approach is to make that situation as irrelevant as possible by *isolating* the insomniac under investigation—for example, by putting her on her own in a lab, even though she usually sleeps in a house full of people, with a dog by her feet.

The desire to find universal laws that apply to sleeplessness as in the natural sciences leaves little scope for the idea that insomnia may not have a single cause, such as an error with the brain, but may instead be caused by several factors, which are different for every person.

Another issue that comes to light when you try to understand insomnia within the template of the natural sciences is that every study has to be "value-free." You can only establish facts if your beliefs or cultural background are excluded from this process. But how do you carry out value-free research into a mental or emotional *disorder*? What we consider a disorder is always based on what we all deem disordered, i.e., not *normal*. And norms are never value-free and universal. What is normal here is exceptional somewhere else, and what deviates from the norm now was once very normal. Value-free measuring, the way you can measure the temperature at which water boils, is by definition impossible when it comes to disorders.[3]

Let's take nighttime waking, for example. If you wake up night after night at around two o'clock and can't get back to sleep again quickly, you have a sleep maintenance disorder. At least, that's how we see it today. But until halfway through the nineteenth century, that was the norm. For centuries, Westerners had a "first sleep" and a "second sleep," terms that found their way into around thirty languages. It was completely normal to go to bed around ten and sleep until around one. After that would be "the watch": a nightly parenthesis of one or two hours in which people discussed their dreams, had sex, or maybe did some household chores. They would then have their second sleep, until it was daytime.[4]

This way of sleeping came to an end during the course of the eighteenth and nineteenth centuries. The industrial revolution, which was in full swing, called for continuous production and therefore a new rhythm. The introduction of bright, affordable, artificial lighting also meant that bedtime could easily be pushed back. Evening entertainment was made available to the urban elite in theaters and cafés, while regular people started working longer hours in shops and factories. Thus, a single, efficient block of sleep became the norm. And sleep in two blocks? That became a disorder.

If the way you sleep is given a label like that, the next time you wake up at night you will think: oh no, there you go, that's my disorder. Why on earth am I put together in such a way that I toss and turn every night while normal people just sleep? You take a disorder like that as a given, something definitive and inevitable. But that's not the case. A disorder is actually a rule that says: you ought to be sleeping *this* way, not *that* way.

When I realized this, I thought: hey, I'm onto something here. Where I previously found myself up against a wall with my problem, I now felt a bit of freedom to move. A little hole in the dead of night, a beginning I could pick away at. If I lie awake at night, I sometimes say to myself: look, that was my first sleep, now it's "the watch." I'm not sleeping badly per se, I'm just doing it seventeenth-century style. And if I manage to bear that in mind, the second sleep follows on its own.

Another example of the dominant, mechanistic view of sleep can be found in the repeated warnings about blue light.[5] That hue of light is thought to interfere with the production of the hormone melatonin, thereby disrupting the diurnal rhythm of your biological clock. A whole industry has been built around that idea. Filters on your glasses, apps, and special lights promise to protect you from your screen's evil blue eye.

However, the danger that blue light poses to your sleep is actually questionable. The light intensity that a tablet or telephone emits is probably much too small to influence your internal clock. A screen emits approximately eighteen lux, whereas you would encounter around a hundred thousand lux outside on a sunny day. Even at full brightness, your smartphone doesn't reach the threshold value for light that is disruptive to your body clock. Leaving your phone alone at night therefore appears to make *no* difference to the concentration of melatonin in your brain; scientists who specialize in the biological clock put a big question mark over all blue light warnings.[6]

At the same time, it won't come as a surprise that using your phone a lot, especially just before bedtime, doesn't help.[7] But is that because of the light? Or what enters your mind *via* that light?

By constantly talking about blue light, the connection between smartphones and sleep appears to be physical: light waves and melatonin. As a result of this, we soon forget the more integral effects of our use of smartphones. A blue light filter doesn't filter out the unrest your phone causes, for example by disconnecting you from your environment, or inviting you to fill every spare second. I will return to this later.

For now, the following conclusion suffices: the purely scientific, "value-free" view, which focuses on physical phenomena and the brain, has its limitations when it comes to insomnia.

In the following hours I would therefore like to look beyond the brain. At the context in which that brain is conditioned[8] and at the world to which it responds: a world that is not free of bias and in which we are not impartial—and in which we sometimes have feelings so strong they keep us up.

Hyperarousal doesn't really explain why I am so persistently awake and an oversensitive stress system doesn't explain where my stress comes from. These explanations may have come from a type of science that focuses exclusively on what is tangible, measurable, and controllable, but for me as an insomniac, they have the opposite effect. For me, neurons and graphs aren't tangible or controllable.

On the other hand, people and things *are* measurable. I measure my insomnia on the basis of the bright yellow earplugs beside my bed, which are getting increasingly grubby. Or by the extent to which I have to bribe myself with chocolate to get through the day. And if I try to figure out *why* I am not sleeping, I don't think of melatonin, but of the man lying beside me, or not lying beside me. I don't think of blue light, but of the red text on my bank statement. Not of hyperarousal, but of the young boy, barely seven years old, who I saw hyperventilating during a climate march. Those are the things that carry meaning to me, which I can see and touch, and to which I can relate. And that is where, as an insomniac, I decided to start looking for explanations.

17:00
YOU FEEL MORE THAN YOU FEEL YOU DO

EARLIER, I WROTE that emotions such as worry and anxiety play a major role in the development of sleeping problems. That didn't surprise me, but it wasn't an insight I could do anything with either. I often had absolutely no idea what I was feeling when I was lying awake. If there were certain emotions preventing me from sleeping, I didn't know what they were. I did feel *something*, but it was a vague, shaky feeling: a sense of turmoil I couldn't put a name on. It was like lying awake because of banging sounds coming from the other side of your bedroom wall, without knowing who or what was causing them.

Our consciousness does not provide a full overview of what's going on inside us. If you had presented me with this statement, I would have undoubtedly underlined it. Yet I still tacitly assumed that I genuinely knew what was going on in *me*.

Every individual has impulses and motives of which they are not aware. I had to go looking for mine. All sorts of things were floating around in the shadows of my cranium: if only I could find out what.

Those twilight zones of the mind, and how to illuminate them, are the subject of the upcoming evening hours.

I used to have a poem by the great Dutch poet Judith Herzberg on my bedroom wall. It is called "The Way."[1]

> *The way you sometimes get to a room, not knowing why*
> *and then have to figure out what you were after,*
> *the way you take something out of a closet*
> *without feeling around for it and only after you hold it*
> *know what you were looking for,*
> *the way you bring a package somewhere*
> *and when you leave are startled, feeling too light,*
> *the way you wait for someone, fall madly in love*
> *for a second with anyone passing, and still go on waiting.*
> *The way you know I've been here once, what was it about,*
> *until a smell comes back to tell you what,*
> *the way you know whom to be careful with*
> *and whom not, whom you can lie down with—*
> *that's the way animals think, I think,*
> *the way animals know the way.*

I was reminded of this poem, about thinking the way an animal thinks, when I read a book by Paul Verhaeghe. He is a professor of clinical psychology and psychoanalysis at Ghent University; a man with a friendly face and a considerable catalogue of titles to his name. His most recent, *Intimiteit* (Intimacy), is about the complex intertwining of body and mind.

In that book I stumbled over the following sentence, "Our thinking is not limited to our consciousness." That confused me, as how do we think outside our consciousness?

Thinking is the same as consciousness, is it not? And your consciousness is the only part of you that thinks?

Not at all, Verhaeghe said, when I asked him that question in a quiet café in Ghent. "Take animals; most animals think, but without our form of consciousness. What is striking is that we *can* think from our consciousness. Humans are probably unique in that respect."

Thinking subconsciously, like an animal. It was a thought that stuck with me and that I wanted to get my head around, human as I am.

The idea of subconscious thought processes was first put forward by Sigmund Freud, the Viennese psychoanalyst who coined the term "the subconscious."

Verhaeghe is quick to mention Freud's name when I ask him about subconscious thinking. He speaks somewhat protectively of the bearded scholar. "Freud's idea of the subconscious was ridiculed at first, only to be later embraced by science under a new name. We now call it 'autonomous thinking' or 'implicit thinking.' But it actually boils down to the same thing. If we look at the brain's activity from a medical and neurological point of view, it never seems to stop. The brain is *always* active. Our consciousness just doesn't always keep up with it."

For a while scientists thought that the brain could be switched on and off like a machine. It was on whenever information was coming in from outside, or when a task needed to be completed. The rest of the time the brain was off. They believed there was either focused, consciously controlled activity, or virtually no activity at all. In the latter case, the brain was probably on standby. This neutral mode was certainly useful, researchers thought, because if you carried out a PET scan on that resting brain, you would get a zero mark against which to compare measurements from an *active* brain.

But when brain researchers did scans like that in the 1990s, what they discovered left them stunned. The zero point didn't seem to exist. Even if you aren't ostensibly doing anything, don't claim to be thinking about anything, or are daydreaming or sleeping, the brain lights up in PET scanners like a metropolis during rush hour. Some parts of your brain even display more activity in this default mode than when you are actively busy doing something.

Perhaps your mind is still busy dealing with unresolved issues in this period of "rest," without you noticing. Your brain goes over anything ambiguous, as if it has a label on it that says, "You are not done with this yet."[2] This could be anything—for example, something new, puzzling, or intense. You don't notice any of this contemplation yourself.

But can it keep you up?

In principle, unconscious (or autonomous) thinking is more or less separate from conscious thinking, Verhaeghe explains. However, there are times when they interact. "At night, you might wake up because a certain autonomous thought process is forcing itself on the conscious mind. For example, if I am working on the intensive final stages of a book, I might wake up at three thirty in the morning with a brilliant idea that ties together the loose ends from the previous day. Problems can be solved at night, as you often discover in the biographies of scientists or artists."

Mary Shelley, for example, said that the idea of Franken-stein came to her in a dream, and the periodic table of the elements is the fruit of Dmitri Mendeleev's brain simmering away at night. The tune of "Yesterday" came to Paul McCartney at night too. Verhaeghe explains, "There is obviously a certain relationship between conscious, focused thinking and unconscious, unfocused, autonomous thinking. You see the two come together at a certain point, and that is the point at which we wake." It is as if autonomous thinking is knocking at the door: hey, I know I'm not meant to disturb you, but you really have to see this.

This kind of thing can also happen during the day; that's the form I am most familiar with myself. You might have spent a while grappling with a problem, to no avail, and then not thought about it for a while. You washed the dishes, had a shower, let the dog out. And then suddenly, as if someone else finished off the work for you, an answer came tumbling into your consciousness as if from nowhere.

In short, your mind never rests. Not during the day and not at night. Even if you don't realize it, all sorts of things are going on. Outside your conscious mind, and without your control, a type of thinking is still taking place.

Apart from unconscious thinking, you can also *feel* without realizing it.

By way of example, Verhaeghe describes the incredible phenomenon of the "non-fearful panic attack." This term was coined when it came to light that one in three people with a panic disorder didn't experience fear. Their body may be displaying all the signs of a panic attack—heart palpi-tations, shortness of breath, dizziness, nausea, trembling, the inability to sleep—but fear? No, they aren't afraid, they wouldn't know what of.

"Someone can be anxious or depressed without consciously being aware of that," Verhaeghe explains. "Their body shows that something is wrong, but they don't know it themselves."

Being in a panic without realizing it; how is that possible? How can you have an emotion so strong your body goes completely out of control, without consciously experiencing that emotion?

"Above all, what that means is that we have an incorrect interpretation of what emotion is," Verhaeghe says, smiling. Emotion, he explains, mainly takes place in your body. It is a type of tension to which you respond in a physical way: you brace yourself, your muscles tense up, your heart rate increases. But it's perfectly possible that you don't notice any of that. "If you say: I feel fear, I feel desire, I feel anger… It means you are feeling it *here*," Verhaeghe says, pointing to his forehead. "Prefrontally. With your conscious mind. In other words, it means you have felt the tension in your body *and* interpreted it as an emotion."

However, this tension doesn't always get translated into an emotion. Often, feelings remain unconscious—your body temperature rises, for example, or your hands get clammy—but because you're not aware of it, those feelings don't reach your brain. That's how I once convinced myself that meeting up with my ex didn't bother me. When I sat down opposite him in the café, I congratulated myself on my nonchalance, only to realize afterwards that I had been gripping the edge of my seat with my hands the entire time. It was only when

I saw the damp imprint they left on the suede that I realized how terribly nervous I must have been.

In psychology, "affect" is the umbrella term for feelings, moods, and emotions and their observable manifestations, whether they are consciously experienced or not. Each conscious emotion starts as an affect, Verhaeghe explains. "A mental awareness *may* subsequently be linked to such an affect. Only when that happens is it called an emotion." A red face, for example, is an affect until your brain consciously assigns a label to it ("I am blushing... I am embarrassed").

Emotions relate to affect the way the zoo relates to the jungle. In the zoo of emotions, every creature has its tag, but outside everything rustles about in the bushes anonymously. Affects are emotions without an enclosure or name.

And that's the norm, not the exception. Verhaeghe comments, "The ability to consciously perceive emotions, to name and discuss them, is an evolutionary luxury probably reserved for humans." A dog with its tail between its legs probably isn't thinking "I'm scared."

But this kind of awareness isn't a given for humans, either. Funnily enough, whether you have access to it depends on your degree of animal, physical intelligence. In other words, whether you succeed in translating affects to consciously experienced emotions depends on how in touch you are with your body.

You therefore have a constantly active, autonomous brain: you think more than you think you do. And your body is full of unconsciously perceived emotions: you feel more than you feel.

When I hear Verhaeghe speaking like this, I can picture myself lying in bed, heart pounding, as I formulate the next day's shopping list in a state of high arousal. I often think: it *can't* be the buttermilk and mushrooms that are keeping me up. But usually nothing else comes to the surface in my nocturnal maelstrom.

If we can think and feel outside our consciousness, there is perhaps a reason why I am doing horizontal pirouettes at night after all; a reason that is hidden in that twilight zone of my mind that isn't visible to me.

I ask Verhaeghe if you could explain sleeping disorders as the result of intense feelings whereby the affect has not become known.

"Yes," he says.[3]

I therefore make it my mission to find whatever is sneaking around in the bushes. I have been trying to ignore the rustling sounds, but it is difficult to set aside thoughts or feelings you don't even know you have. It is time to confront my unconscious thoughts and feelings, my affects, my twilight zone. But how do I do that?

One way of learning how to better translate affects to emotions is by training your body awareness. Lots of meditation exercises (and other methods, like Feldenkrais therapy, yoga, and mindfulness practices)[4] start with you closing your eyes, sitting still, and noticing what you can feel in your body (muscle tension, warmth, cold?). You can also do this without meditating, by focusing on what your body is *doing* during the day: Do you start sweating when you receive an email from your boss? Do you suddenly feel exhausted when you have to think about money? Do your clothes smell of sweat

at the end of one day more than other days? What is happening in your body when you sit down at your desk? Give
it a try for a day.

Therapy offers another way of learning to feel what you
might secretly be feeling. A psychologist or psychoanalyst
is skilled at coaxing things out you didn't know you knew.

Sometimes an outsider who happens to ask the right
questions can be enough.

A journalist, for example, once asked me what the meaning of life was. (He was writing a series on this topic for the
Dutch newspaper *de Volkskrant*.)[5] That's not something I
stop to think about on a daily basis, and my own response
surprised me. I said that I saw life as a thin thread, stretched
out from A to B, running above a complete void. (Oof!) You
spend your life connecting this thread to more places, and
tying it to others, in the hope it becomes a piece of fabric:
something that can give you stability. Life doesn't have a
meaning of its own, I said; a safety net of meaning only
exists if you make it yourself.

When I read the interview back later, I thought: whew,
how grim! Obviously I feel like I'm going through life like a
tightrope walker. I hadn't been explicitly aware of the anxiety my answer revealed: that I am balancing precariously,
and that unfortunately there isn't a safety net like the one
there used to be in the sleeper train.

I started wondering whether there was a link between my
insomnia and the precarious, wobbly feeling of the tightrope
walker, which came to the fore during sleepless nights. That
feeling is not an invitation to let yourself fall—into sleep or
whatever else.

But should I really be linking the meaning of life to my tossing and turning? Was that not reading too much into a physical ailment? And what's more: Isn't the question too large to solve? I wanted a quick fix, as I needed sleep *immediately*. However, after reading the interview in the paper, I couldn't shake the feeling that the trouble I had "letting go" at night did, in fact, have something to do with that lack of a mental footing. In order to take this intuition seriously I needed scientific backing. I shall take a closer look at this in later hours.

Before that, I want to look into the third way of becoming aware of hidden emotions.

Alongside training body awareness or finding someone who asks the right questions, there is another route to the twilight zones of the mind: the much-hailed, semi-mythical pathway of the dream.

18:00

DREAMS AS
A WAY TO ACCESS
EMOTIONS

SIGMUND FREUD called the study of dreams "the royal road
to a knowledge of the unconscious activities of the mind."
But even well before his time, dreams were seen as a form of
communication. They were thought to contain a message
to the dreamer.

Opinions about who or what was sending that message have changed over the millennia. In various cultures
dreams were, and still are, seen as something powerful
and even sacred, with the source coming from outside the
person, from the supernatural. Prophets met their god in
their dreams, while ordinary people received messages and
premonitions.[1]

For a long time, dreams had not only a spiritual, but
also a practical meaning. The Greek doctor Hippocrates,
for example, asked his patients about their dreams as well
as their physical symptoms, because he believed that these
often contained the key to medical diagnoses.[2] And in
nineteenth-century England, the predictive dreams of the
victims and witnesses of a crime were still often used as part
of the police report.[3]

Nowadays we rarely think of dreams as a source of higher wisdom. Instead, they are seen as a product of our own mind. The dream is no longer a signal from above, but an electrical trace in the brain, made visible by new measuring equipment.

This equipment has generated a vast amount of knowledge since the middle of the last century. It has been shown, for example, that in REM sleep, the phase in which most dreams are reported, various regions of the brain become very active, such as the parts of the brain responsible for visual and spatial perception, as well as the motor cortex, which controls movements. The hippocampus, which is involved in memory, also lights up, and the brain's emotional centers (the amygdala and the limbic system) are strikingly active: 30 percent more so than when you are awake. But when it comes to asking what all of this activity means, a brain scan has nothing to say. "Nothing" was therefore the prevailing answer.

In the 1970s, a new theory about dreams emerged: dreams are a coincidental by-product of the brain. Researchers had discovered that the chemical balance in the brain changes when you sleep. This change, they thought, triggers reactions in the brain stem: signals that are generated by pure coincidence and through a physiological process. The poor brain, confronted with this chaos, then does its best to concoct a somewhat logical story from all of that neural "noise."

To put it simply, dreams didn't mean anything. By this time, Sigmund Freud's theory that dreams were a way of expressing suppressed, unconscious impulses had been thoroughly discredited. So much so that all references to Freud's work and to the subconscious had been removed from the leading manual for psychiatry, the *Diagnostic and Statistical Manual of Mental Disorders* (DSM).

The meaning dreams sometimes appear to contain, as well as the fact that they sometimes seem able to predict events, was all attributed to chance. Think about it: you dream four or five times a night, and that adds up to such a huge number of dreams over the course of a lifetime that it is hardly surprising, purely on the basis of probability, that one pops up every now and then that is similar to a later real-life event. Nothing superhuman, just a matter of statistics.

Dreams have never managed to overcome this disenchantment. Lots of scientists still regard their contents as meaningless today.

The fact that the contents of dreams are dismissed as meaningless does not mean that today's sleep researchers don't assign any functions to them at all, or rather to dream sleep or REM sleep.

If you prevent animals or people from getting REM sleep for a while, it won't take long before all sorts of things start going wrong, particularly in psychological and emotional terms. Memory declines, people report feeling sadder and more anxious, and they perform worse on all sorts of tests. People who don't get any dream sleep are less able to read facial expressions, for example, and interpret them more negatively than necessary. As a result, they behave more timorously and less socially.[4]

The theory is therefore that dream sleep is vital for emotional health: a type of nocturnal self-therapy for the brain. The dream *itself* is a by-product of this, or perhaps an instrument. Dreaming about a drastic event, for example, appears to help you process it or emotionally prepare for it. People who dream about their divorce fare better emotionally a year later than those who don't, and students who dream about an exam in advance perform better, on average, than those who don't.[5]

How is that possible? The prevailing explanation points to the absence of certain signalling chemicals in the brain during REM sleep, such as noradrenaline, the neurotransmitter that works like an adhesive in your brain and that is associated with stress. As we learned in earlier chapters, noradrenaline is *not* usually released during dream sleep, which gives connections in your brain the opportunity to disappear. It is possible that this allows your mind to process emotional or traumatic situations in a dream, after which they are less emotionally charged, or to "try out" exciting prospects in advance, in a chemically safe environment. Think of REM sleep as a period in which the theater of the mind is covered with rubber tiles, so you can give all sorts of acrobatics a go without breaking anything.

If that's true, dreams would be able to provide something other than self-therapy: playfulness and creativity. That idea mainly came about when Robert Stickgold, sleep researcher at Harvard, discovered that people who are woken during REM sleep gave looser, less obvious answers during a word-association task. His theory was that because the parts of the brain responsible for logical thinking are less active during this phase of sleep, the brain is quicker to make illogical, more surprising connections. A certain type of intelligence is under way, but a much looser one. It usually generates rubbish, but sometimes it lucks out.

Stickgold therefore compares the dreamer to a venture capitalist. Logical thinking can be seen as a safe investment of your brainpower, which generates a safe, albeit small profit. On the other hand, when you are dreaming, "you are making bold investments [with your mental energy]. If that produces rubbish most of the time—very well; you are dreaming all night long anyway. If 80 percent is a waste of time, and in that one remaining hour you generate a useful association that you wouldn't have made otherwise, that's a great outcome."

While the dream was once a bridge to a different world, or a divine message, now it is a risk investment. The function we assign to our dreams offers a portrayal of mankind in miniature.

Outside the lab it is more difficult to believe that dreams are simply neural noise, a mental pinball machine or a coincidental by-product of brain maintenance.

You might have had a dream at some point that knocked you off your stride for a while after waking up. Every now and then I wake up with an overwhelming feeling of sadness because someone has died, and I am so convinced of what I have just experienced that it takes a while for me to realize I was dreaming.

These are dreams that tell me how afraid I am of things I never worry about during the day. Time and time again I see my boyfriend disappear, drown, or shrink until he fits inside a snail's shell. Other people or animals I care a lot about suffer similar fates. There are other things my brain is forever dishing up for me at night too, each time in a different form, like mashed, reheated food I refused to touch the previous day.

Over the past years it has struck me just how often I would dream about dictatorial figures. When flicking through the channels on my personal dream TV, Xi Jinping, Trump, Erdoğan, and Putin kept popping up on every channel in the form of GIFs with flaming tongues and little stars for eyes. One time they were working as gigolos in a brothel for lonely people. Another time, Viktor Orbán introduced a ban on all weather phenomena apart from snow and sun, just in time for my camping holiday.

If you were to ask me during the day if I am seriously concerned about the end of liberal democracy, I would say, "No, there's no real risk of that." If you were to ask my dreams the same thing, they would have a different answer. The question is whether I ought to take that other answer seriously. Can my dreams tell me something about what's keeping me up?

If there is one branch of science that sees dreams as useful, it's psychiatry.

Sigmund Freud thought there are certain thoughts you won't allow to become conscious—for example, because they are too shocking. You suppress these thoughts during the day, but you need to release control of your consciousness in order to sleep. That's when they get the chance to reveal their true colors.

But if every dark thought simply surfaced from your subconscious, it would cause you to jolt awake. According to Freud, that's why "dream work" takes place. Whatever has been suppressed surfaces, but only after it has been disguised and transformed into a somewhat bizarre story that looks innocent enough not to wake the sleeper.

When I ask Paul Verhaeghe to explain what exactly is going on during dream work, he says, "Freud's main theory was that each dream is the fulfillment of a wish. An expression of a hidden desire. Lots of people are familiar with that notion, but what people may not be familiar with is what Freud added to that: the dream is the fulfillment of a wish, *and the ultimate wish is to continue sleeping.* The dream helps make this possible." Dreams are intended to enable you to continue sleeping, by putting a new spin on the troubling musings of your subconscious.

Sometimes that goes wrong. The dream mechanism may fail, for example because the material from your subconscious is too intense. The result is a nightmare. "According to Freud, that is a failed dream because it wakes you up, which is completely the opposite of what a dream is meant to do."

Verhaeghe's British colleague, the psychoanalyst Darian Leader, also refers to Freud's theory in his book *Why Can't We Sleep?*, stating that dreams make topics that would usually keep us awake compatible with sleep. This process can go wrong in the form of nightmares, but also in another way.

Leader explains, "If the disturbing elements are just too strong or too present, we forgo sleep altogether." In other words, if too much is going on, the mind would rather let sleep bypass it completely than risk giving up conscious control.

But even without sleep, the mind is not completely immune to whatever is going on in the gray zone of our subconscious, Leader writes. You might be familiar with the special phenomenon of nocturnal panic: inexplicable profuse sweating, clammy hands, and the conviction that something is about to go terribly wrong, which overcomes you at night, and which you are unable to explain to anyone during the day, not even yourself.

According to Leader, the anxiety and distress we feel when lying awake in the middle of the night are our "experience of the proximity of the subconscious." It is as if we can hear the storm hidden inside us raging behind the thin wall of our conscious thinking.

If that is true, the topics processed in our dreams are precisely the same ones that impede our sleep.

I can well imagine that to be the case. There are things that, insofar as I *know*, no longer bother me—for example, an ex with whom I still have plenty to discuss. I genuinely never think about him during the day, and haven't spoken to him in years. Yet for months my autonomous thinking presented me with a dream a couple of times each week in which he would appear. Sometimes we would get along; usually he was angry. In the end I asked around for his contact details.

Dreams can bring unconscious affects into the conscious mind via an impressive story, thereby helping make our implicit thoughts explicit. By this I am *not* referring to simplistic dream interpretation with "dream symbols" and "dream dictionaries" that say things like "If an eel appears in your dream, you have a fear of commitment."[6] The content of dreams, and the associations that play a role in them, are far too personal to make such general statements.

However, there is a type of dream interpretation that is supported by modern dream research. Freud's theory may have been ridiculed by science for some time now, but many of his ideas are returning in a brand-new guise.

For example, the idea that whatever is "suppressed" resurfaces in dreams has been repackaged as the "dream rebound effect." Researchers established that test subjects who were not allowed to think about polar bears during the day were much more likely to dream about these animals than members of a control group who had been encouraged to think about them. It has also been shown that people who strongly suppress their emotions are more likely to dream about emotionally charged experiences.

Another sign that dreams are deeply rooted in the psyche is the fact that people with psychological problems very often have recurring dreams. These dreams only stop when the underlying cause or conflict is resolved. Because of this link, some doctors regularly ask depressed patients about their dreams. If these dreams are violent and feature lots of death and suffering, this is seen as a warning sign that the person is suicidal, and that action is needed *now*.[7]

Psychiatrists are not the only ones who use dreams as a source of knowledge about their patients. Doctors who deal with physical health as opposed to mental health are sometimes interested in dreams too.

In *Why We Dream*, a history of dream science, the American author Alice Robb includes a number of anecdotes about patients who first become aware of their illness in a dream. She mentions a Russian psychiatrist who collected sixteen hundred dream reports from patients in the hospital where he worked. He derived from them that the patients had often had nightmares about injury, blood, dirt, or hospitals immediately prior to displaying symptoms of an illness. Some patients dreamed specifically about the part of the body that was later affected.

The famous British neurologist Oliver Sacks includes similar anecdotes in his work, for example in *Awakenings*, his book about "sleeping sickness": an epidemic that swept the world at the start of the twentieth century. Anyone who contracted sleeping sickness became lethargic, succumbing to a slowly advancing paralysis that ultimately left the patient trapped inside their own body. They ended up unable to move or respond to the world. Sacks, who treated patients with sleeping sickness for many years, reports in his book that some of them had suffered from intense nightmares just before their symptoms manifested. These sometimes seemed to predict the fate they later suffered. The future patients dreamed that they were frozen or locked up in an impregnable castle that was exactly the same shape as their body, or that they had been turned into a statue: all prophecies of what was to come.[8]

The dream as a prophecy of a physical ailment only seems strange or implausible if you assume that the mind and body are two separate things as opposed to a continuous whole.

If you are now interested in the nocturnal products of your mind, the question that arises is: How to dream?

Even very bad sleepers sleep a bit, and a bit of sleep is, in principle, enough to dream. The challenge is to remember that dream. If you want to practice, you can put a notepad beside your pillow and before you go to bed, say to yourself: *I will dream and I will remember that dream.* The more you think about it during the day, the more likely you are to succeed. Even reading these lines is a good start.

It appears as if dreams can be more or less invited: the more you listen to them, the more they will tell you. That's my experience at least. I rarely remembered my dreams. But since I immersed myself in the myths and science surrounding them, I started remembering at least one dream almost every night. I still often have crystal clear, cinematic dreams today.

For real fanatics, the next step is lucid dreams. Those are dreams in which you are aware that you are dreaming. Some people become so skilled at this that they claim they can control their dreams: flying, saving the world, working things out with that ex. And all of that while fast asleep. The first step towards dreaming lucidly is to repeatedly ask yourself during the day: *Am I dreaming now?* Once this question becomes automatic, it may occasionally pop up in a dream, and if the answer is yes, you can start controlling it—at least if you don't wake up from the shock of your first successful lucid dream.[9]

If you don't usually dream very much, there are a couple of very simple steps you can take to dream more. First, don't take any substances that are known to suppress your REM sleep, the sleep phase in which dreams mainly occur. Drinking alcohol, for example, is a very efficient way of hampering your dreams. The same applies to sedatives and tranquilizers (like benzodiazepines). Antidepressants are also known to impede dream sleep. The fact that the use of them is so widespread is therefore also bad news for our dreams.[10]

However, the most significant killer of dreams could well be the alarm clock. This is because REM sleep is not evenly distributed throughout the night: the lion's share occurs in the early hours of the morning, in the last two hours of your sleep. If you get up early, after about six hours' sleep, you may only be losing around a quarter of your hypothetical eight hours' sleep, but you are surrendering 60 to 90 percent of your dream sleep.[11]

Our hectic schedules are therefore detrimental to the part of our sleep richest in REM. In other words, the more focused we are on "living the dream," the less time we have to actually dream.

Recounting a dream is seen as a literary faux pas. Most writers are acutely aware of the famous warning: "Tell a dream, lose a reader."[12] A dream is seen as a very ostentatious way of saying something about a character. But when it comes to your own life, the significance of dreams is best embraced.

I have personally never based a major decision solely on a dream. The inferences I make tend to be more modest: I might, for example, dream that I have lost someone dear and then decide to call her the next day (it was high time!). Or I might dream about forest fires and droughts and the next day determine that I will no longer travel by plane. It is only when a dream topic regularly recurs that I really pay it any notice.

Dreams like this function like a personalized Rorschach test, helping me to ask myself a critical question from time to time. What's on my mind? What's bothering me? And am I paying it enough attention during the day? Sometimes that helps me address a nagging concern. Other times that concern is too big and beyond my powers.

Fairly recently I dreamed about an illness you could pass on to someone else at will. I was at a lively party and knew that one of the young men there had the illness. I kept a nervous eye on the room. Every now and then, one of the other guests' heads would light up and a white ring would pop up around it. I was surrounded by beautiful young men and women—actually still girls—who were happily chatting away unsuspectingly. Suddenly, I twigged that the man with the illness was infecting all the women who refused to pay him any attention. "Touch me," he said, and just before I woke up I saw that his right hand was a scorpion.

When the pandemic began I read lots of reports about "COVID dreams." They often featured masks, floating viruses, and impending physical contact. So many people reported experiencing a high number of unusually intense dreams that researchers started collecting dream reports. A major, far-reaching change that affects many people can evidently be seen reflected in the way in which dreams are collectively experienced.

The most famous example of this are the dreams collected in reports by the German Jewish journalist Charlotte Beradt between 1933 and 1939. As Nazism gained power, she asked her fellow Berlin residents about their dreams. Whether a neighbor, the doctor, or the milkman—they all seemed to dream about similar things: bugged telephones, Aryan declarations, houses left without any walls. The nightmares were often more intense than the political reality appeared at the time. The people foresaw or apprehended which disasters might come. An ophthalmologist dreamed about concentration camps, and when he saw that he was wearing nice, shiny boots, and was prepared to collaborate, he broke down in tears.

However, collecting these dreams was a risky business. In order to keep them safe, she concealed what they were actually about. "Arrest" became "flu," "Goebbels" became "Uncle Gerhard," "the party" became "the family," and so on. She sent them to acquaintances abroad in this encoded form, before fleeing Germany herself in 1939. Only decades later did she publish her report under the title *Das Dritte Reich des Traums (The Third Reich of Dreams)*.

What Is Keeping You Up?

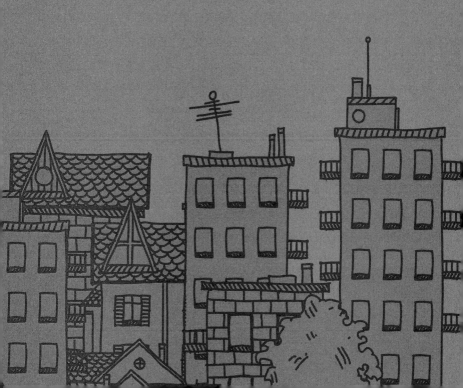

19:00
CONTEXT

IF OUR DAILY LIVES CHANGE, our nights change too. We may start dreaming differently, and we may even collectively spend more time lying awake.

There is a strong connection between the way in which a society is organized and the mental health of the people in that society. The World Health Organization clearly states that mental health is shaped by social context.[1] The United Nations claims that the dominant biomedical view of mental disorders is misleading, and that social context deserves much greater attention.[2] These statements relate to anxiety disorders and depression,[3] but there is no reason why they shouldn't apply equally to sleep disorders. After all, anxiety and depression are very closely related to insomnia.

It is therefore time to focus on another question. Instead of "Which part of the brain is involved in insomnia?," I would like to find out: Which circumstances are involved?

I have already mentioned the role of emotions in sleep problems. Those emotions do not exist in a vacuum; they usually come about as a response to specific circumstances. Your financial situation, for example, can have a major impact on your mood, as can your living situation and the people around you.

In the following section I would therefore like to look at a number of factors *outside* your brain that influence your sleep. I will focus on what I consider the most fundamental, practical ingredients in a person's life: money (or the lack of it), time (and the feeling of time pressure), place (your physical environment and how you relate to it), and others (the people around you).

This brings us to the question that probably led you to pick up this book in the first place. The usual sleeping tips aren't working; you still regularly find yourself lying awake or your sleep isn't restful. So what *can* help? In order to answer that question, as a new night approaches, I would like to take a close look at the building blocks mentioned, at the role they play in sleep, and at the practical ways in which you can adapt them so you can actually improve your sleep. However, there's a problem: it is not always possible to transform these building blocks. You cannot always change circumstances entirely on your own.

COVID-19 has made that very clear. There are also many other things that jeopardize our sleep but that cannot be controlled through personal interventions. Just think, for example, of the climate crisis, which will make sleep more and more difficult as temperatures continue to rise.[4] Or a financial crisis that causes widespread stress; rising unemployment rates; or increasing work pressures. Think of increasing social division, racism, or war. There's not much you can do about any of these as an individual. They are societal issues.

Your direct context, or personal life situation, isn't necessarily easy to change either. Some readers may be tied to a certain place, have time-consuming obligations, or need to live close to a hospital. Different readers will have different limitations. For that reason, what follows are a number of suggestions you can apply where possible, and which—even if they cannot be applied literally—identify an avenue that may be worth exploring. Taking those suggestions as a starting point, everyone can explore what is possible for them. And that is often more than they might think.

20:00
MONEY

LET'S START MUNDANELY, with money, since wealth and poverty help determine how likely you are to lie awake at night.

The relationship between money and sleep is a complex one. On the one hand, sleep is a billion-dollar industry, which is also experiencing substantial growth. The market data company Statista estimated that the global sleep industry is currently worth 432 billion dollars, and predicts that this figure will rise to 585 billion dollars per year by 2024.[1] In comparison, the global book industry is worth around 110 billion dollars per year.[2]

There is money to be made out of our broken nights. Research company McKinsey writes that "There are billions of dollars stuffed into the mattress!" in a report gushing about the "wide range of attractive market opportunities" tied to the fact that "more than one in three Americans does not get enough sleep."[3]

And that sleep industry is not just about pills and supplements. One of the more creative ways of earning money through other people's sleep is Pokémon Sleep, a game that was planned to be released in 2020 but had still not appeared at the time of writing. You might be familiar with its predecessor, Pokémon Go, where players walked around trying to catch Pokémon creatures that appeared on their phone screens at specific real-life locations. The miles they covered in the process were converted into extra points. Pokémon Sleep will reward you in the same way for the number of hours slept: the more you sleep, the more virtual creatures and imaginary gadgets you get. But the people who are really getting rich while you sleep are the owners of the game. The ad players see when they wake up is worth a lot of money, and although it is not yet clear exactly which user data will be collected, it's easy to see how intimate information about how well or badly millions of players are sleeping can be turned into money.[4] Pokémon Sleep promises to help players sleep, but above all it is helping itself.

Our yearning for sleep is a gold mine for others. The commercialization of sleep comes in many guises: from little cushions designed to help you relax by breathing slowly, to electric hairbands designed to stimulate slow sleep brainwaves, and machines that produce calming static adapted to your own brain's activity. From YouTubers pretending to be your boyfriend as they soothe you to sleep,[5] to glasses that filter out artificial light, to supersonic mattresses. For anyone with money going spare, technologically enhanced sleep is already attainable.[6]

The promises all these products make sound wonderful. But also a bit ominous. A pulsating cushion designed to mimic slow breathing is advertised with the slogan: "Sleep well, live well."[7] A mattress: "Sleep. Live! Every hour counts."[8] "You lose about one IQ point for every hour of sleep you lose." You don't live as long either, the consumer is informed.[9] "Sleep better, live longer. The better your sleep quality, the longer you live."[10]

There's a lot at stake, that much is clear. It is actually a matter of life or death. In their alarmist ways, manufacturers echo researchers like Walker, who likens a lack of sleep to "slow euthanasia." Well then, sleep tight!

But do all these smart sleep devices actually work?

Unfortunately not. Perhaps they help people who already sleep well to relax, Eus van Someren says. "But the problem is that sleep gadgets are usually marketed at insomniacs. Take the Somnox, that bean-shaped cushion that detects your breathing rate and helps you relax by slowing it down. A fantastic idea, but not for insomniacs. Those are people whose senses are all very sharp." After all, they are characterized by hyperarousal. "So as soon as that cushion changes rhythm, they wake up. It becomes yet another disappointment: something else that doesn't help. The same applies to Fitbits and other tracking devices. These work quite well for good sleepers, but are pretty much useless when it comes to insomniacs."

And it is insomniacs, in particular, who are willing to dig deep into their pockets to try and get that unattainable sleep.

I have never tried smart gadgets like that myself. I may have been tempted to test out a breathing cushion, but I had enough trouble paying the rent. There were times when I would regularly hear the "payment declined" beep at the checkout. I found it so stressful that the items on the conveyor belt gradually gave way to sedatives. Those were located on a really long shelf with the sign "Sleep and Rest" above it, so I could simply add them to my shopping list: milk, butter, a sack of potatoes, and thirty lots of sleep and rest.

Only the pills didn't help, which led to the confusing conclusion that you may not be able to buy sleep, but it is a matter of money nonetheless.

Counting sheep is more relaxing if you don't have to count pennies. In general, the less money you have, the more likely you are to experience sleeping problems. If you line up five Dutch people from poor to rich, the first is almost twice as likely to have disturbed sleep as the last one.[11] In the U.S. too, low income often goes hand in hand with poor sleep. For instance, an American man who makes $10,000 to $15,000 a year has about 88 percent more chance of having sleep complaints than one who makes $50,000 to $75,000.[12]

Income is closely related to educational level,[13] and there, the same trend applies: the lower the level of your education, the more likely you are to sleep badly. Conversely, the higher your level of education, the less likely you are to have sleep problems. Dutch people with a lower level of education are almost twice as likely to experience sleep problems as those with the highest level of education.[14] A Brit who hasn't completed secondary education is twice as likely to suffer from sleep problems as one who has.[15] And an American woman who hasn't finished high school has about a 64 percent greater chance of developing sleep complaints than one who has finished college.[16]

Seeing how money and sleep are linked, it's relevant that wealth is often unequally distributed among people of different ethnicities, too.[17] It isn't just education that impacts how much money you're likely to have in the bank; race is tied into the mix.

In the U.S., for instance, the net wealth of an average white family is nearly ten times greater than that of a Black family.[18] The average Black and Hispanic or Latinx households earn about half as much as the average white household.[19]

It isn't surprising to see corresponding sleep disparities, too. Black Americans on average have less "deep" NREM sleep than whites; both sleep duration and quality are lower in people of color than white people.[20] For instance, Black Americans report very short nights—less than six, or even less than four hours a night—two to two and a half times as often, respectively, as white Americans.[21] Black Americans and Latinx people also disproportionately work night and early morning hours, which harms their sleep.[22]

Although differences in wealth and the comfort it buys explain a lot of this racialized "sleep gap," the experience of racism also plays a significant role; more on this in chapter 23:00.

There are also gender-related differences that correspond to income inequality. Women[23] all over the world consistently report sleep problems more often than men. In the Netherlands, they do so more than one and a half times as often.[24] A meta-analysis of international studies shows that women run about 58 percent more risk of having insomnia than do men.[25] Smaller studies also consistently show a gender difference; for instance, more than a quarter of American women suffer from it, compared to less than a fifth of American men.[26] Almost one in three Dutch adolescent boys suffer from disturbed sleep, whereas more than half of girls do.[27] Canadian women report sleeping badly "all of the time" more than twice as often as Canadian men.[28]

Researchers in the past have supposed a hormonal cause. But it might be more logical to find a different explanation. The gender difference in sleep problems *halves* if you take income into account. In other words, if you compare men and women with the same income, the difference in sleep problems between genders is suddenly half the size. This means that it is mainly the lower socioeconomic status of women that explains their additional sleep problems.[29] In the Netherlands, four in ten women are not financially independent[30] and the income gap between men and women amounts to three hundred thousand euros over the course of a working lifetime.[31] Women in the EU on average earn about 14 percent less per hour than men.[32] In the U.S., in 2020, women earned 16 percent less than men earned per hour.[33] The racial and gender pay gaps combine spectacularly for Black women, who in America make only 63 cents for every dollar made by a white man.[34] In the U.K., women in 2022 were paid 90p for each pound earned by men.[35] In the long run, of course, those differences add up. Not a particularly restful thought!

Why is there such a strong correlation between money and sleep? Money isn't soporific in and of itself;[36] but there are many practical reasons as to why you might sleep less if you have less money. Perhaps you live in a noisy room as opposed to a spacious, well-insulated apartment. You may not be able to afford healthy foods and be ill more often.[37] You probably worry about paying your bills.[38] (It is hardly surprising that people who don't know where their next meal is coming from struggle more to fall asleep and stay asleep, and that they wake up earlier than those who know they have enough to eat.)[39]

You also have less choice when it comes to work; if you don't have a lot of money, you are less able to defend yourself against the demands of employers, such as irregular working hours, holding several jobs at once, or working night shifts.[40] During the height of COVID, this also meant working jobs where you were exposed to the virus.

The types of work available also partially explain the influence of education level on sleep. Less-educated people are more likely to work night shifts or irregular hours, which make a set sleeping pattern extremely difficult.[41] The World Health Organization claims that night shift work is "probably carcinogenic," based on the evidence that it causes severe sleep disturbances, which in turn may lead to cancer.[42]

Night shift work is hardly ideal, but no work at all is even worse. Almost 40 percent of those without paid work have sleep problems, compared to 25 percent of those with a regular job.[43]

To summarize: whereas financial insecurity robs us of our sleep, economic security is *good* for our sleep, and for our mental health in general.

There is one experiment that has made that particularly clear: the famous "Mincome" experiment with universal basic income carried out in Canada in the 1970s. All residents of Dauphin, Manitoba, a town affected by poverty, as well as some randomly selected residents of Winnipeg and rural Manitoba, received an income for three years without having to do anything in return. It was not a huge sum of money, but enough to make ends meet. The residents were followed by a research team, who carried out all sorts of measurements and calculations.

The results were sensational. Three years of financial security was enough to see a significant difference. People with a basic income needed to go to hospital less often—by a difference of around 9 percent—and they went to their doctor significantly less often too. It wasn't because they were suddenly immune to a sprained leg or the flu; the reduction in doctors' visits, for each and every one of them, was due to the fact that they had fewer mental health complaints: less anxiety and depression and fewer sleep problems.[44]

After three years of basic income, the experiment was cancelled: Canada got a new conservative government, which saw no future in the experiment and put an end to it. However, the basic income experiment has since been repeated in various places, such as Barcelona, where approximately a thousand households from deprived areas received about 1,600 euros per month between 2017 and 2019. The findings were similar to those from Canada. They revealed that Barcelona's residents who were able to rely on a stable income were 10 percent less likely to develop mental disorders. They slept better too.[45]

So, forget sleep hygiene, the list of superficial sleep tips for those who can afford expensive mattresses, quiet homes, and relaxation regimes. What would do our sleep (and our health in general) a world of good would be to tackle poverty and inequality.

That's all well and good, you might be thinking. But what does this mean for the insomniac in practical terms? You can't simply conjure a higher salary, and universal basic income is still a utopia.

A couple of years ago I tried to crack this nut myself. As mentioned, I often struggled to make ends meet, and my automatic reflex was to work more: write more, speak at more events, write more essays, more columns. It wasn't the better jobs, but the better-paying ones that took precedence. I didn't stop to think that there could be another way: by spending less. I didn't exactly have a lavish lifestyle, so didn't feel like I could save much this way.

That changed when I left behind my room in Amsterdam to live without a fixed address for a while. I spent a spring, summer, and autumn traveling around with my backpack. I usually camped; sometimes I would stay with friends or do some housesitting. The idea was that by living as cheaply as possible I wouldn't have to take on as much work. That would give me time to think about my next book.

During those months I started seeing time and money from a different perspective. In order to have time I had to make sure I took on as few jobs as possible. And to be able to take on as few jobs as possible I had to be frugal. Wild camping for a week meant I could write one fewer piece that month, so would have more time. I kept track of all my expenses, only went to a café if I needed Wi-Fi, and got creative with the camping stove.

In short, I was economical. Not with my time, because time costs money; but with my money, because *money costs time*. The more I published, the less time I had for the puzzle I wanted to solve.

Of course, I wasn't the first to discover this. There is a whole movement based around the ideal of living as frugally as possible in order to "buy" your freedom: the FIRE movement. FIRE stands for "Financial Independence, Retire Early."

I read about this school of financial independence via the blog of a middle-aged Canadian who goes by the name of Mr. Money Mustache. After a brief office career, he gave up work. All of his time is now free time. He cheerfully writes that he has achieved this "simply by living a lifestyle about 50 percent less expensive than most of our peers and investing the surplus in very boring index funds."

He started his blog out of frustration. He was fed up with hearing his friends and former co-workers complaining about their money troubles and saying how they would love to work less. "These comments were generally made over expensive pints of microbrew at a restaurant," Mr. Money Mustache writes. According to him, most people live ridiculously expensive lifestyles and are then "baffled when they [have] no money left over to buy their own freedom."

If you want to amass that ransom money, it might seem logical to strive for more income: work more, or borrow money. On the contrary, the FIRE movement puts the emphasis on less. Spend less. It is actually very simple: if you don't need much, you soon have enough. And you are "financially independent" more quickly. That works in two ways. The less money you spend, the more you can save if you do work, and the longer you can get by with your savings if you (temporarily) stop working or start working considerably less.

In my case, "needing less" was mainly a matter of paying less rent. Because even though I was already living in a relatively cheap room with a shared kitchen and bathroom, my living costs were by far my largest expense.

The same applies to most people. For the average household, living costs are the biggest expense. Furthermore, we are spending more money on our accommodation now than a couple of decades ago, relatively speaking.[46]

When I started researching how to reduce my own living costs, it seemed there was only one solution: to move house. House prices can differ significantly depending on where you live, and my boyfriend and I put these differences at the forefront of our house hunt. In the end we found an old, rather dilapidated house in the Morvan. It's a beautiful, sparsely populated area in Burgundy, in central France, where thousands of houses are abandoned and therefore relatively cheap. If we had stayed in Amsterdam, we would have been able to buy a hundred-square-foot garage for the same price.

So now we are living in our new, old house in Burgundy. Shopping, electricity, and insurance are our biggest expenses. And with it a huge weight has been lifted from our shoulders, and from our agendas.

I wouldn't have been able to take a step like this at an earlier stage of my life, and there will certainly be times in the future when I am bound to a certain place again. I am aware that many people won't have the luxury of simply picking up and moving to a place where the living costs are low, perhaps because they are tied to a certain job or need to care for a relative.

But there may be other options, and it is worth considering where, exactly, your money is going. If you ever worry about money, or if you would like to work less, you can try the following: download your deposits and withdrawals from your online banking statement, put them in a spreadsheet, and sort them into various categories: living costs, travel costs, shopping... What are your biggest expenses? How could you decrease them? If you spend a lot of money on takeout coffee, start taking your own in an insulated mug. Cook for the people you usually eat out with. Or make a gift for someone's birthday instead of buying one.

Of course, this is a strategy you have to adapt to your own needs. You might notice that you are saving a few dollars a week on coffee, but you are also missing out on the best part of your day. Or that keeping too close an eye on your finances stresses you out. None of these things are good for your sleep. The idea is to simply reduce your financial pressure by needing less money. I have saved myself a lot of stress, and therefore also sleeplessness, by no longer having to work towards the monthly deadline of an Amsterdam rent.

It can also be insightful to find out how many hours you have to work to cover each expense in your spreadsheet. How? Simply take your total deposits and divide this figure by the number of hours you spend doing paid work: that's your hourly wage. It is important to remember to take account not only of the hours on your contract, but also the time needed to commute, to do your hair or makeup, to send a quick reply to your boss in the evening, and to recover from something you might be reluctant to do. If you don't divide your total income by the number of working hours on your contract, but by the number of hours you *actually* devote to your job, your real hourly wage ends up being significantly lower. You can use that figure to convert your expenses from the currency of dollars into hours.[47] That tells you how much time a certain expense really costs.

You get a better impression of how high your expenses really are if you see how many living hours they demand, week in, week out. You may realize you are losing twenty hours a week simply to pay your rent or mortgage. Hours that you are trading for the pleasure of a noisy one-bedroom apartment. A good deal?

From this point of view, every expense becomes a question of "your money or your life."[48] And that can shed a different light on costs that initially seemed entirely reasonable. That new phone, is it really worth a hundred hours of your time?

We often say that "time is money," but money and time cannot really be exchanged. With some effort, you can often get ahold of more money once yours has run out, but once your time is up, it's game over. Because time is irreplaceable, it is in fact a harder currency.[49] As a result, it is not especially wise to spend all your time amassing money. It makes more sense to spend all your money amassing free time.

21:00
TIME

WHEN COVID-19 CRIPPLED PUBLIC LIFE, our world was turned upside down. While lots of people suffered from stress and sleepless nights as a result, others thrived.[1] The daily commute was eliminated; you just had to look presentable in front of the Zoom camera. You no longer accidentally found yourself window-shopping on the way home from work. Those who weren't suddenly burdened with the responsibilities of home schooling found themselves with a lot of time on their hands. "All of a sudden, I've got so much time," I kept hearing people say. And, for those with a secure income, there was also suddenly so much *calm*. "It's only now that I realize how busy I always was"—I must have heard about twenty different versions of this same sentence. It was usually followed by something along the lines of, "It's a breath of fresh air, to be honest." When the second wave broke out, and the world closed down again, a friend of mine even sighed, "I'm glad, really, because I'd been starting to get overworked again."

I burst out laughing. But it is actually perverse that it takes an emergency situation to keep us from flying through our days at breakneck speed.

What would you do if every day unexpectedly had more hours in it? Would you finally start reading more, walking more, cooking more; would you spend that time looking for a better job or finally start thinking about the house move you didn't have the energy for before? How would your evening look, and would that make a difference to your night?

For quite a few people, their lack of sleep is a direct consequence of a lack of time. In a survey carried out in Amsterdam, three in ten men and as many as *half* of women reported that they didn't have enough time to sleep. It is therefore not especially surprising that 80 percent of those surveyed were unsatisfied with their sleep. The sleep doctor Kristel Kasius, who commented on the study, stated that a lack of time was one of the main causes of sleep problems among her patients. "I see lots of young people in Amsterdam who don't have the time to relax and sleep. There are not enough hours in the day for everything: family, career, sports, parties, and so on. Sleep has to be squeezed into the limited time that is left over."[2]

Not having the time to hit the hay is one thing, but a lack of time can also indirectly eat away at your night. Even if you spend enough hours in bed, you may not be able to get to sleep because you have spent the whole day in a race against the clock.

Hectic working days often go hand in hand with disturbed sleep.[3] If your work pressure is too high—or you have too many tasks and not enough time to complete them— research shows that you often sleep less *and* worse: you have trouble falling asleep and staying asleep, and the sleep that you do get is less restful.[4] Even the prospect of something stressful is often enough to make people sleep less, sleep less deeply, and wake up more often.[5]

People whose jobs require them to rush around doing several things at once while being constantly interrupted are significantly more likely to suffer from psychological complaints and sleep problems.[6] According to studies, time pressure is one of the main risk factors for the development of sleep problems. Having to work at top speed is not only a physical challenge, but a psychological one too, and this mental pressure again results in worse sleep. A hectic work pace is therefore much more likely to go hand in hand with serious stress and exhaustion.[7]

To summarize, time pressure plays a role in the development of sleep problems.[8] And that is important, because time pressure is currently seen as the biggest stress factor overall at work.[9]

Perhaps you are familiar with that sense of hurry you can't shake after you have spent the whole day going about your business at a hundred miles an hour: even if you no longer need to race around, you can't slow down. You power walk, speak quickly, eat or hold on to your bike's handlebars with one hand while replying to an email with the other. It is as if you have set off a metronome whose tempo you can no longer change. People who have established such a pace have a long braking distance at night.

As I am trying to articulate why rushing around during the day is so detrimental to my sleep, I think of the canisters of polyurethane foam I recently used to fill in some cracks in the loft of my home. You might have used it yourself: viscous blobs come out of the canister and expand extremely quickly. You know what they are going to do, but the force with which it happens takes you by surprise. If you use polyurethane foam with too great an "expansion factor" in a space that is too small, the foam continues to expand and further splits apart the crack you had hoped to seal.

In the same way, lots of events in my daily life tend to expand in my consciousness, with disturbed nights as the result.

Impressive encounters or exciting work events often need more space than the moment in which they occur. They expand like cognitive or emotional polyurethane foam. Even when I have already processed them, they keep popping up again. What did X mean when she said that? Did I express myself properly in that meeting? I should have said something else. And the expression on Z's face when he told me... Especially at night, all sorts of memory fragments come to the surface. I underestimate their expansion factor; perhaps for me it is simply higher than for other people (or perhaps I become hyperaroused more easily). All I can do is wait patiently until these impressions have unfurled and taken up all the necessary space in my mind before I can hope for some sleep.

I always had the tendency to set aside the exact number of hours or minutes needed to get through everything that had to be done in a day. And certainly no more. Once I had finished one thing, I would move straight on to the next, pronto, because time was of the essence. Thanks to my smartphone, I didn't have to waste a single minute; you can even reply to your emails on the toilet.

I have had to learn to factor in a bit of free time between all the different tasks. I might use that time to go for a walk, or simply sit on the sofa with my dog and let my fingers glide through his fur as my mind goes through the day. The effect of that has been massive. The different tasks are now like cookies spaced far enough apart on the baking tray; they can still expand, the way experiences often do, maturing and rising in a warm-blooded body. And as a result, I no longer have to try to organize the mishmash of my day at night.

That's all well and good, but how do you find more time? Not everyone's schedule is as flexible as a writer's. However, it can still be worth looking for the wiggle room in your agenda. A good place to start is by finding out exactly how long you spend on each activity. Which things cause you the most frustration and stress, and which things are you always happy to have done? In other words: What feels like a waste of time, and what would you like to devote more time to? This will give you an overview of the surplus and deficit in your time budget.

For the majority of people, savings in the category of "paid work" can be most beneficial. As mentioned earlier, I gained time by living more frugally; by moving somewhere where the cost of living is lower, I no longer have to write X many articles per month to pay the rent.

This move also put an end to a string of coffee dates. Requests I once found difficult to decline are now impossible to accept. Sometimes that's a shame, but usually, to be honest, it's just fine.

There's a whole host of things that take up more time than you would like. You will be familiar with the examples: spending half an hour deciding what to wear; going to the supermarket without a shopping list and wandering around aimlessly with a half-full basket; picking up your phone to check the weather forecast and somehow ending up spending an hour scrolling. You can consciously take measures to overcome frustrations like these.

This leads me to my final tip: don't rely on good intentions. If you really want to change something, you need to find ways to compel yourself to do so. I only spend less time on Facebook now that I have hidden my profile, and I consistently spend more time walking now that I have a dog who starts scratching at the door whenever I threaten not to bother. Habits are so stubborn that a good intention stands no chance without a helpful compulsion. You could fill a whole bookcase with psychological research to back that up.[10]

However, there is an exception to this rule. If you alter a major aspect of your life—for example, by moving house, changing your job,[11] or ending a relationship—everything is up in the air for a while. The routes you usually take, your mode of transport, your routine: you will have to reorganize all of these things. As a result, for a brief while you will have the opportunity to adapt those stubborn habits associated with your old life to your new one. It doesn't take long; after about three months you are already set in your ways again and the opportunity has passed.[12] So if, in your attempt to improve your sleep, you want to change one aspect of your life, be aware that that also offers scope for changes in other fields—and that you can gain time there too.

22:00
PLACE

THE MOST RESTFUL THING you can do with your time, if you are to believe the self-help articles and coaches, is to be in the "here and now." If you know how to find your way there, you can leave all your stresses behind. All you need to do is get rid of "later," "earlier," and "elsewhere," and simply be where you are.

I never really worked out how to do that, despite my best efforts. There is something funny about "here and now": the more I studied it, the less I believed I would ever find peace there.

My "now," for example, didn't really mean much. I can place an order, do my admin, check my finances, or watch a favorite show at any time of day or night. There was always something open in the city. What does the time on the clock actually mean, apart from how long I have been lying awake?

My "here" didn't mean much either: a small south-facing room, which became unbearably hot as soon as the days started getting longer. I was living there because I had to live somewhere, but there were plenty of places I would have rather been. Luckily for me, I could go virtually anywhere via my phone screen or laptop. "Here" is a corridor with a thousand doors in it that are always ajar.

When I was a child, "here" was still a relatively hermetic place. You could leave it, for example through books, but those escapades were clearly defined. We watched television after dinner and a film on a Sunday morning. We were only allowed to read after we had finished our homework. But on the whole, we were usually simply "here."

Today, being half-present is the norm. When I used to look out the kitchen window of my flat in Amsterdam, I would see people staring at screens as they walked or cycled past. They were physically moving, but they were mentally already elsewhere. "Here" has become completely porous. Here *is* somewhere else.[1]

Some cities, such as Bangkok and Xi'an, have built separate smartphone lanes for pedestrians and cyclists who want to use their smartphones on the go. Seoul is trying to reverse this trend by painting the words LOOK UP on the sidewalk in bright yellow block capitals. Many other places are adapting to the new reality. From Melbourne and Tel Aviv to Singapore: "zombie" pedestrian signals are being installed in the sidewalk that you can see flashing without even having to look up from your smartphone.[2]

The built environment is adapting, little by little, to our absence. It is hard to think of a better confirmation that the "here and now" is just an empty husk. It is therefore hardly surprising that we are restless, and in search of a (digital) place we find more interesting.

Imagine how different life would be if your environment played a key role. If everything around you was relevant to your life. In order to get an impression of what that might be like, I read *Change in the Village*, written in 1912 by George Sturt, a wheelwright from Surrey in the U.K.

Sturt made wooden wheels, as his family had done for generations. But the country life in which those wheels belonged started to disappear around the end of the nineteenth century. His village was nothing special, he wrote: an inconspicuous hamlet in a narrow valley. The soil was poor, as were the people. However, for generations they had known how to get by, in a hundred different ways. They didn't need a lot of money, because they mainly lived off what they could make or grow themselves: their vegetables and crops, their clothing, their wheat, bread, and wine, their honey, and their haystacks. The fact that they succeeded at being so self-sufficient was not only due to the vegetable garden that belonged to each house. There was also the common—the big patch of communal ground on the slopes around the valley. That's where they let their livestock graze, chopped wood for building, cut peat for their bread ovens, and so on.

Then something happened in the village that was happening all over the country: access to communal land was restricted. The common was privatized, partitioned, and sold off. And with it, the farming system that had worked for centuries collapsed, "like an arch from which the keystone is removed."

Without the common and the resources it provided, people suddenly had to buy everything, from firewood to cattle feed. They had to earn money, so found paid work. The women got jobs cleaning the villas of new, wealthier residents; the men sought work in the construction of a railway line, or they delivered coal. The lucky ones found jobs in the village, constructing pleasure gardens or tennis courts for the wealthy. The unlucky ones spent their days in a quarry. Over time, Sturt saw more of his fellow villagers descend into apathy. A key part of their lives seemed to have disappeared.

Of course, village life was also difficult before the loss of the common. But still, Sturt wrote, there was something precious about it. Life may have been difficult, but it had a certain value. It was *interesting*.

First of all, the days were varied. Depending on the season, in the morning you might have picked hops for a neighboring farmer, at the end of the afternoon you might have returned home to feed your pigs or make wine, and in the evening you might have tended to your vegetable garden. All of these activities required skill, experience, and knowledge. As a result, people were proud of their work: of the wine they had made themselves, or of the bread made from their own wheat. A type of pride that couldn't be found later, in the coal mine.

What's more, the fact that the work was so deeply rooted in the place where it was carried out made the environment *itself* interesting, right down to the smallest detail. After all, the villager's livelihood depended on it. That's why "[He] knew the soil of the fields and its variations almost foot by foot; he understood the springs and streams; hedgerow and ditch explained themselves to him; [...] the local chalk and clay and stone, all had a place in his regard—reminded him of the crafts of his people, spoke to him of the economies of his own cottage life; so that [...] the timber he handled when at home called his fancy [...] to the landscape [it] came from."[3]

All of this meant that a villager didn't just inhabit his village; he was part of it, and it was part of him. He *belonged* there, the same way all the other indigenous animals did. And just like for a hedgehog or a thrush, everything that happened to his habitat was of importance to him.

Keep that hedgehog in mind, and then think of the people with their phones. They are walking on a part of the sidewalk that has been specially set aside for them, where they can stumble around without having to look up. That is the difference between a world with a lot of "here" and one with very little.

Sturt's book portrays the transition from a world in which every object means something to one in which most things don't affect you. Food, for example, is nowadays simply food: you buy it, you consume it, that's the extent of your connection with it. A grass field is someone else's lawn, not somewhere for your goat to graze. The village, which once formed the heart of the surrounding hills, is now an insignificant satellite, entirely dependent on the nearest big city.[4] Nothing it has to offer is actually interesting for the people who live there; everything is shrouded in a veil of insignificance.

"I shall be told that, after all, this is mere sentiment," Sturt writes. "But, then, half the comfort of life proceeds from those large vague sentiments which lift a man's private doings up from meanness into worthiness."[5]

That's all well and good, but how can we lift our everyday activities up into worthiness? Or, to put it more precisely, how can we reconnect with our environment?

The old French house my boyfriend and I moved into barely had a kitchen. The counter was a plank of wood resting on wobbly stone blocks and the antique sink leaked, so we decided to rip it all out. We knocked down walls and tiles, chiseled, and painted. Meanwhile, we waited for our IKEA delivery, which never turned up: our hamlet proved too difficult for the delivery driver to find. We spent months cooking on a precarious camping stove and washing up in the tiny sink beside the shower.

I now have the best kitchen in the world. Well, the walls are conspicuously crooked, the sealant is a bit messy in places, and the handles aren't quite in the middle of the drawers. But if I look at the counter, which may not be perfectly varnished, I can picture the truck that delivered it. It was too big to navigate the narrow streets, so we had to carry the counter across the whole village—much to the amusement of our neighbors—with our puppy at our feet, tail wagging. From chipping away at stubborn grout in the depths of winter to long mornings sanding in the spring sunshine: I've invested months of my life in this kitchen. If someone were to offer to demolish it all and replace it free of charge with a perfect, professional, luxury kitchen, with neatly sealed edges and symmetrical handles, I would indignantly decline.

There is a name for this reaction: the IKEA effect. This explains why people appreciate a cabinet they have put together themselves more than the same one bought pre-assembled. People are even willing to pay more for something they have to invest time and energy in, for example a teddy bear from a make-your-own-bear kit, which would be cheaper ready-made. This still applies if the result is obviously flawed, or even a resounding failure in other people's eyes. Lopsided or not, the handyman themself will discover qualities in it that no one else can see.[6]

According to psychologists, the IKEA effect is a fallacy, or irrational behavior. But is it actually that irrational? Or is it irrational to dismiss the human tendency to become attached to things as abnormal? People who don't become attached to things are psychopaths.

Those same psychologists explain that there are countless irrational mechanisms of attachment. The "mere exposure effect" describes the tendency to evaluate things more positively simply because they are familiar. Whether they are people or nonsense words, if you have seen them once before, you are more likely to attach a positive meaning to them.[7]

Or the "endowment effect," which refers to the way people value an object they already own more highly than they would if they were to buy a new version of the same object. In an experiment, people had to indicate how much they would be willing to spend on a coffee mug. Not a lot, it emerged. Another group was given the same mug and then had to indicate how much money they would want for it. Suddenly, the same mug had more than doubled in value. In short: the fact that something is yours—or even that you have just held it—is enough to increase its value.[8]

Regardless of whether you have assembled something yourself or are simply familiar with it, the need for attachment is extremely important. People are willing to spend their Sunday mornings traipsing around flat-pack furniture stores just so they can turn screws into pre-drilled holes when they get back home again. Even a badly assembled piece of furniture made from chipboard is lifted "from meanness into worthiness" if you have assembled it badly yourself.

That is sentimentality for you. But half the pleasure of life comes from such sentimentalities.

Incidentally, you don't have to go to IKEA to benefit from the IKEA effect, and you don't have to do a major renovation either. DIY can take place on a smaller scale too: by cooking, brewing your own ginger beer, or pouring your own candles. Things a thirty-minute YouTube tutorial can teach you. You can benefit from the endowment effect too: see it as an excuse to sew a new zipper into that old, tattered jacket you are secretly attached to, however scruffy it might look.

Making things yourself is just one way of assigning new value to your surroundings. Another thing that could help you reach that infamous "here and now" is a different kind of "here."

For example, I never had the space for a vegetable garden in the city, whereas it is now an important part of my daily life. It makes various aspects of my environment relevant all at once: the weather, the type of soil, the various critters that turn my kitchen waste into compost... The bee stings my boyfriend got when working in our flowerbed had a sweet aftertaste thanks to the honey the beekeeper at the edge of the village gave us as a gift.

Actually, I am aware of the value of everything here, even the water from the tap. The entire village relies on a single natural spring, with a single reservoir. When it's gone, it's gone. We water the young lettuce plants with the dirty dishwater, and no rain means no bath. What's more, we are so isolated that you can't just go and buy something. The people who grew up here automatically try to find anything they might need locally. If the street is dug up for the installation of new cabling, they immediately turn up with wheelbarrows, ready to use the excavated earth to level out their gardens. If one neighbor has a bit of curtain fabric left over, someone else repurposes it as a seat cover.

It didn't take long for my boyfriend and I to follow their example. The old windows we replaced with double glazing became a greenhouse, thanks to a few planks of wood and some nails. And while I would have previously gone to a garden center to get a trellis for our peas, it is now only natural to simply cut down a few willow branches from the woods. That saves money and an hour's drive.

The "barter economy" isn't something hip here, but simply the way things have always been. Before we knew it, my boyfriend and I were also part of that culture: our Wi-Fi password for your drill, a cake as a thank-you for helping dig out the pond, and if I can borrow your chainsaw, you can have some of the wood.

All in all, it is much easier here to be where I am, without getting sucked into the digital vortex. And that leaves me feeling calm.

But even if you are tied to a rental apartment in a city, you can still seek ways to fill the place you live with more meaning, and to connect more with your physical environment.

Green oases, for example, can also be found in cities. When I lived in Amsterdam, I would often see an old woman with a headscarf walking through my neighborhood. She would be collecting sweet chestnuts or picking herbs I never knew were edible or otherwise usable. For anyone interested, urban nature has more to offer than you might think. You can grow a surprising quantity of herbs, lettuces, or vegetables on a balcony, flat roof, or windowsill. Your city might have a community garden where you can rent a plot; or you can simply adopt a small bed around the foot of a tree.

It makes more sense for urbanites to find their "here" not so much in the natural environment, but more in the social or cultural environment. You might feel more rooted in your neighborhood if you bypass the supermarket that looks the same everywhere, and instead build up a relationship with local shops. Even if you then risk being reprimanded because they "haven't seen you in a while" (like my boyfriend in the corner store). Or you might make a good guess in the annual "how much does the pumpkin weigh?" competition at the grocer's and end up having to lug the monstrosity back home. I delighted in the grocer's friendly "Hello neighbor" whenever he saw me after that.

Another option is to make a point of going to your appointments by foot, instead of by bike or car. (That immediately creates a bit more space between the cookie dough on the baking sheet.) Borrow a guidebook from the library or take a historical tour around your own city. Volunteer as a buddy for a lonely neighbor. There are all sorts of ways, some practical and others less so, in which you can add more meaning to your environment. Perhaps you can think of some others.

So far, I have focused on what you can do to feel better-rooted to the place you live. I have not yet mentioned another aspect of this place, although the topic seems obvious to someone who has moved to the countryside: how *green* that living environment is.

If you are a chronic insomniac, there is something to be said for switching pavement for trees. Shinrin-yoku, or "forest bathing," as the Japanese call it, has been shown to quickly lessen feelings of depression and anxiety.[9] There are indications that living in a green area can help you get a good night's sleep. Even simply having "nature" (such as a park, forest, or beach) close to your home has been shown to significantly reduce your risk of poor sleep.[10] That positive effect is not dependent on socioeconomic factors, and holds true even if people don't use that space to exercise more. Just looking at the chlorophyll seems to help.[11]

Looking *and* moving may be even more helpful; going for a walk in green surroundings appears to aid sleep. A study from Japan—where around *one in five* people suffer from insomnia—showed that insomniacs slept better and longer if they had taken a walk through the forest at lunch.[12] In cities, the number of trees also makes a difference when it comes to sleep. The bigger the canopy in a certain neighborhood, the more likely residents are to say they sleep well.[13]

And sleep is not the only thing that benefits. A longitudinal study among five thousand Brits showed that the mental health of those who moved to greener areas improved significantly and that these effects were sustained. They were less anxious and less depressed, compared to those who moved to less green areas.[14]

To put it simply, green is good for your mental health. And that also applies explicitly to your sleep.[15]

To some people the suggestions in this chapter might seem to go too far; others would convincingly argue they're not nearly going far enough. One of those people is Roslyn Von Senden, a Kalkadoon woman from Mount Isa, Queensland. She is a community worker and serves as cultural advisor and sleep coach for Dreamtime, Australia's first

Indigenous youth sleep program. Dreamtime was launched in 2021 by the University of Queensland to address the sleep gap between non-Indigenous Australians and Aboriginal Australians and Torres Strait Islanders, who sleep less and worse than their white compatriots. This is a pattern also seen in Indigenous people in New Zealand, the U.S., and Canada, with the sleeping problems compounding and being worsened by other mental and physical health issues.[16]

Speaking to me by telephone, Roslyn Von Senden starts by sketching the issue she sees at the core of her community's problems: the loss of Aboriginal ways of knowing and doing.

"I live in a rural area, desert-like, dusty, with hot, hot heat. It gets so hot here during the day that traditionally we only hunted very early and late. During the day, people would sit around telling stories about what they knew, resting, breast-feeding children, doing artwork like rock art representing what they had dreamed about. Activity and rest would be guided by the rhythms of the land: by the evening star, which is the first to come up at night and the first to go down in the morning; by the timing of the animals who in the late afternoon were going for water. People didn't recognize just four, but eight seasons, sometimes more; and we would know what food to find where at every one. When spiders wove their webs very close together, we'd know it would be a cold winter. Our people still know these things. They know the wood of the gidgee tree burns stably for a long time; they know what materials to use to insulate from the heat."

The result of this way of life, living sustainably off the land, was that "every element from every piece of sand and dirt and grass was used for *something*. All had a purpose."

This has changed radically with the violence and dis-possession inflicted by colonization. Von Senden takes me, at breathtaking pace, through the history of battles, forced displacement, and Aboriginal babies taken away to be placed with white people, and the intergenerational trauma that still resonates today.[17]

It has become hard to carry on life in the old way, because the context has changed. "Imported animals like cattle are damaging the land and waterways; mining has raped the land, and vegetation has suffered. We've lost a lot of the sea-sonal knowledge, like when to burn out the land so plants would grow back after the rains." But the Western way of life also isn't working out for many Indigenous Australians, she says. "Many people have employment difficulties, they face poverty, overcrowded housing, unhealthy foods, alco-hol problems, and heavy care burdens for their families. It's hard trying to live as an Aboriginal person in a Western context. Not everyone can. Under these circumstances it's not surprising that sleep is a big problem."

Von Senden is one of the people trying to conserve and pass down ancient Aboriginal knowledge. When I ask her what she teaches her community to help them sleep, she immediately says: "Get out in nature. Listen to the different sounds and smells, observe the movements of animals... And leave your technology at home. If you have music play-ing you won't be hearing the bush, you won't feel the pattern of harmony. Look at the stars. Be embraced back into that environment."

She talks about traditional bush medicines which help to calm you, like eucalyptus and lemongrass, but when I ask for specific tips and strategies for sleep that she shares with the young people she works with, she seems to sigh at my short-sightedness, saying: "We don't just go out there for a little bit so we can sleep. Getting back on country, reconnecting with the tradition and the culture: all that is one. One wholeness. Being at bush is who we *were*. You can feel the urge in you."

The urge, she explains, is "to get away from this crazy world that's making you sick. Get to the real stuff. Tell yarns, fish, sit at the river, make a campfire. Just the smell of smoke is soothing. It's about the whole of it: summertime swimming in bush water, sleeping under the stars and rising with the sun ... If I do that, I feel revived, ready to take on anything and be what I need to be in this Western world. If I don't go—and I haven't been out for a couple of weeks now—I can't sleep at all."

I ask her to describe what she feels when she is away from the country for a long time. "It's a sense of loneliness, because I'm looking at big buildings around me and no sky. It's a funny feeling that something is missing, like when your kids go away from you."

While she is trying to get the message out to her community that sleep is centrally important to health, she resists looking at it in isolation. Her approach is resolutely holistic. Well-being and sleep are about wholeness, she says. "Yes, we now live in this Western world, but we have to balance the two worlds. We have to keep our culture. It's about more than sleep, it's about a whole way of living that needs to be regained. Going home on country is like touching base."

Von Senden talks beautifully about the importance of place in Aboriginal culture, about the havoc that colonial violence, breaking that link, has caused, and the vital importance of reconnecting to it for wholeness, health, and well-being, which sleep can't be severed from.

"Indigenous culture knows many things the West has forgotten," she holds, "resulting in a rootlessness and respect-lessness for our surroundings which are at the core of much of the mess we are in." She gives me a glimpse of how we might approach sleep, health, and indeed life in general, if we were to broaden our view and step outside of the hamster wheel of stress, smartphone addiction, and concrete.

23:00
OTHERS

THE TREMENDOUS SILENCE that falls upon our French village at night is pleasant, comforting, and a luxury—unless I am alone. Then I suddenly feel compelled to lock the door. I know that otherwise I will lie awake listening for strange sounds; what was that I heard coming from the attic?

Sleep is not only closely associated with money, time, and space, but also with others—the people in your life.

Most sleep research is carried out on people lying down on their own in a lab somewhere. By isolating them, scientists can control variables, which makes their research more objective. But it also means that the sleep in a laboratory setting becomes far removed from everyday sleep. After all, people usually sleep in their own beds, and often not on their own. Historically speaking, people have rarely slept alone. Our sleep is therefore social through and through.[1]

We know, for instance, that loneliness can be detrimental to sleep.

The first indications of this, as is often the case, came from experiments on mice. Like people, mice usually live in groups. If you put one alone in a cage for weeks on end, its behavior changes completely. For example, the sleep the mouse gets is strikingly less deep (if you monitor it, you find far less powerful sleep waves). If you give it a sedative, it has less effect than on mice kept in pairs.[2]

It soon emerged that mice aren't unique in this regard. In fact, the same probably holds true for *all* social animals that are isolated, including people. Couples who sleep together sleep deeper than if they spend the night apart.[3] But whether you spend the night alone or together is not the critical factor per se; if you generally feel alone, you are more likely to sleep less well. You typically lie awake at night more often between the fragments of sleep, and your sleep is less "efficient."[4] That is because you constantly wake up very briefly, often so briefly that you don't remember doing so the next day. Scientists refer to these as microarousals.

The lonelier someone feels, the more their sleep is peppered with those brief awakenings. Disturbed sleep in the form of microarousals can even be used as a measurement unit for our sense of loneliness. The lowest rates of microarousals to date were recorded among Hutterites, a closed, religious farming community in the Dakotas that does virtually everything as a group: working, eating, praying, and relaxing.[5]

If loneliness is bad for your sleep, the opposite should also hold true. And it does: people who have active social contact during the day seem to benefit from this at night in the form of better, more efficient sleep.[6]

That is the reason why a stable, happy romantic relationship is seen as beneficial to sleep. A (good) marriage protects you, to some extent, from sleep problems.[7] You might think that having a whole bed to yourself sounds great, but that luxury and the associated peace and quiet do not outweigh the reassuring sense of security associated with sharing a bed.[8] Couples report significantly better sleep than those who live alone. It has been shown that Dutch people in stable relationships are a quarter less likely to have sleeping problems than single people, at 29 and 40 percent respectively.[9] Research among Australian adults showed those in a stable relationship took less time to fall asleep at night than those with occasional or casual partners.[10] Divorced Americans report significantly more sleep complaints than those who are single or married.[11]

On the other hand, a *bad* marriage is often associated with poor sleep. People in problematic relationships report more sleep problems on average than those who are single.[12] A relationship is therefore not a silver bullet. There is also not a simple cause-and-effect relationship between sleep and loneliness. Exhaustion doesn't exactly make you morph into a social butterfly, and sleep problems can also in turn be detrimental to relationships.[13]

I received an indication that my sleep might be sensitive to loneliness in the mail. During my research into the topic of sleep I received a letter from a marketing specialist who had read my articles about insomnia. They wanted to send me a weighted blanket in the hope I would write about it. I was skeptical, but also curious, so a heavy package turned up on my doorstep not long afterwards: a blue blanket into which numerous tiny but noticeable weights had been sewn. It weighed twelve pounds, a good three times as heavy as my trusty down duvet.

I crawled under it, and it comfortingly pressed its weight on me: a small echo of the reassuring feeling I get when my boyfriend stretches out on top of me to "squash" me. The enclosed leaflet referred to "deep touch pressure stimulation." In any case, the intention is to "replicate the feeling that you are being held (like a hug!)." In the same way a baby falls asleep more easily if you put your hand on their chest for a while, the weight of the blanket is supposed to make you feel as if you are being held and gently pushed into the mattress.

It is not especially surprising that there is a market for blankets that imitate a hug. When you ask people how lonely they feel, the conclusion is consistently: very lonely. In 2016, more than four in ten Dutch adults said they felt lonely. One in ten felt very or extremely lonely.[14]

One in five Americans in their twenties and thirties say they have *no* friends: none at all, not even superficial ones. And three in ten are often or always lonely.[15] In Canada, more than one in ten people say they are often or always lonely.[16] One in five Australians rarely or never feel close to people; over one in four feel lonely.[17] After similar reports abouts the "loneliness epidemic" in the United Kingdom, the British government has even appointed a Minister for Loneliness.[18]

Why are we so lonely? Anyone can make a good guess: perhaps our culture is too individualistic and we are too focused on success and possessions. Perhaps, in an era in which jobs last six months instead of for life, we are too busy looking out for ourselves to bother much about anyone else. Perhaps we simply *think* that the rest of the world is out having fun at Instagrammable parties while we are sitting at home alone. Perhaps digital contact, which is gradually replacing physical contact, isn't actually so wonderful after all (a point I no longer have to try and explain since COVID).

Why is there such a strong connection between sleep and a sense of belonging? To answer this question I turn to Paul Verhaeghe, the professor from Ghent University. He likes to analyze society as if it were a patient seeing him for a consultation. I expect he'll have something interesting to say about a society in which we are all lying awake so often *and* feeling so alone. He certainly does: when I refer to the above-mentioned studies, he says that sleep and loneliness are definitely connected, but we need to consider that connection on a more fundamental level.

So back to childhood: Verhaeghe explains that the first sleep problems we all have emerge when we are toddlers, when being left alone to sleep becomes a cause for tantrums and tears. "Trying to get a two- or three-year-old to sleep is almost always problematic," he says. "Why? Because that's when they lose their safe place: their mother or father, their main attachment figure."[19] That's also why they employ delay tactics just before bed: they need to go to the toilet, have a drink, brush their teeth, have just one more story... "This whole palaver is actually just a way of saying one thing: 'stay with me, don't leave me, because I am scared.' This fear hinders the process of falling asleep."

Two things can be deduced from this, he continues. "First, that falling asleep is related to security.[20] You need to feel secure enough to let go of your consciousness. And secondly, that that security is, in the first instance, provided by others." It is only once the child has internalized the presence of the attachment figure, and subliminally "knows" or senses that mom or dad or grandad will come back, that the child is able to sleep alone.

It's not actually any different for adults, Verhaeghe explains. "Some adults also struggle to fall asleep unless they are lying beside someone, preferably their loved one. Because they need that security too."

I recognize myself in what he is saying; I like to sleep best with my boyfriend's arm wrapped around me. When I climb into bed and turn my back towards him, he will say, "Come here then... good reverse parking... a bit further... yes, like that." If I snuggle right up to him, he has my back covered.

The pursuit of nocturnal security from others can take on extreme forms. Verhaeghe mentions a former patient who compulsively sought bed buddies, even for one-night stands, simply so he could sleep. "He would accept the sexual interaction as the price to pay for some shut-eye." And he also mentions a woman who had been a victim of sexual violence, after which she could only get a good night's sleep at her mother's house: she felt too unsafe anywhere else.

Of course, the opposite is also true. Some people can only fall asleep alone, and others can't bear to have someone lying beside them. Verhaeghe explains, "Funnily enough, that's also to do with security. Those people see the other person as a threat; they need distance." Whether we can't sleep alone or can't sleep together—both are down to attachment.

These are perhaps extreme cases. But in a more subtle way, the underlying principle applies to us all: in order to sleep well, we need to feel secure instead of lonely.

Loneliness is not simply a matter of not having enough people around you. After all, it is perfectly possible to feel completely alone in a group or even in a relationship. Like all things, loneliness is a bit more complicated, and touches upon fundamental issues such as how you have learned to relate to the world around you.

In his book *What About Me? The Struggle for Identity in a Market-Based Society*, Verhaeghe writes that we need two things to feel comfortable socially: to belong to something, but also to be able to exist independently. Just think of how we all cheer on our nation's athletes at the Olympic Games, but also how someone might pursue their passion for insect collecting, even if none of their friends understand it. Both ways of being are fundamentally important. Verhaeghe refers to these two processes as "identification" (converging with others, or with the group) and "separation" (being an autonomous individual). They have to be well-balanced. If the group dominates, you feel cramped and restricted. If you are completely on your own, without a group, you feel lonely.

The latter is characteristic of our time—or rather, of our society. Verhaeghe claims that the emphasis over the past decades has been on autonomy and individuality, and therefore on separation. That has its advantages, such as a high level of personal freedom. But it also comes with its disadvantages. Our economic system encourages competition: employees compete for jobs and promotions, self-employed people take each other's work. This mutual competition isolates people and plays them off against each other. As a result, a lot of people are left feeling very lost, and lonely.

"Many of our modern-day problems are related to a loss of purpose," Verhaeghe explains. "It seems that social success and money aren't enough to create a sense of purpose. What we are left with is inner restlessness: Is this it, then?"

There's that tightrope walker again, I think to myself.

That sense of being lost and that inner restlessness, Verhaeghe explains, "are the real reason why we have seen such a huge increase in anxiety disorders, depression, and ADHD over the past years."[21]

And sleep problems? Can they also be attributed to the era of the individual?

Verhaeghe thinks so. Constantly focusing on our achievements and career, which is what society urges us to do, hinders our sleep.

"When people with sleep problems come into my practice, one of the following two things is usually going on: there is something the matter with a loved one (for example, they have a sick child or partner), or they simply can't stop fretting or making plans at night. And if you are too caught up in yourself at night—in your ego, your career, your successes, what is feasible, and everything you need to do—a great deal of stress piles up." In other words, if you concentrate on yourself and your own problems, you end up concentrating tension too. And that keeps you awake.

I could see myself in this portrayal of the insomniac. My nights often collapsed under the weight of an overloaded day. All of the wants, needs, and organizing that the banks of my day could no longer contain overflowed into the night. So there I would lie, feverishly trying to work it all out, to control it all. The early hours apparently served as floodplains for my ambitions, and they were permanently inundated.

But the light Verhaeghe shone on this process was new to me. What I would have described as ruminating about everyday concerns, he describes as ego-building. After all, those thoughts are always concerned with your own position, your own plans, your own growth and career. "The tension you feel in bed at night is due to the fact that as you are ruminating, you are constantly confronted with the fact that you are not there yet, that building your ego hasn't progressed enough."

Falling asleep is precisely the opposite. "You sink into your mattress or the arms of Morpheus; you disappear into a bigger whole. You become one with your environment. But if you are constantly busy with 'me-me-me,' you don't dissolve. Sleeping is disappearing. Surrendering to something bigger."

I would like to learn how to disappear, but don't know how. Surrendering to something bigger: How do you go about that? And what's more, is my generation of Millennials, with our penchant for individualism and going solo, not especially badly equipped for this?

"I fear so," Verhaeghe replies gently. But that's no reason to be put off. Even if society is going in one direction, you as an individual can still go in a different direction. He seems distressed when he adds, "It's hard to explain to young people just how little freedom we had two generations ago. We had a lot less choice, in all regards. Back then, everyone dressed the same, choosing your own gender was inconceivable, the body was sinful, and sex was forbidden. We have so many more liberties today, but we don't take them."

Which liberties does he mean? "We have the choice, for example, *not* to take part in the race for social recognition. Instead, each of us can choose a different type of self-realization, beyond that success story." No one is *forcing* us to adopt the values the world prescribes, he says. We don't *have* to strive for an inflated ego, a Tesla, and a high salary.

Whether or not we continue (nocturnally) building our egos depends on choices that are very much within our power, he says. "For example, how do you treat the people around you? What do and don't you make time for? Which things do you assign importance to? We have a lot more control over those things than you might think. Each of us can decide to reclaim our autonomy, instead of simply joining the procession towards status."

Make more discerning life choices, and don't be afraid to go against the tide if necessary; this sleeping tip was one I had never encountered before.

It's not difficult to guess the direction these choices should take. After all, if we see sleep problems as ego problems and sleeping as surrendering to something bigger, the solution is to be found in less "me" and more "we." If I try to translate what Verhaeghe's told me into concrete tips, I come up with: carefully consider the things that are most important to you in your life. Can you, for example, put your work or personal projects on hold if a friend is struggling? Are you really too busy to take your niece to that theme park she's been going on about for ages? Could you do some volunteer work? In other words, reconsider your priorities. Focus less on your own success, and more on your environment.

You could almost describe it as a social sedative.

I hesitatively suggest this formulation to Verhaeghe; he nods at its self-evidence. "Some advice I often give people is to find a project to work on with at least two other people. Do something together that has a purpose not related to yourselves. *That* is meaningful."

Sleeping is surrendering to something bigger, and that includes during the day.

Incidentally, you don't necessarily need a crowd of people in order to surrender to something bigger. Less "me" or ego? You can get that on your own too. In fact, all activities in which you lose yourself help decrease the stress that is preventing you from sleeping at night.

You might be familiar with the following scenario: you are playing an instrument, cooking, or playing a game, and you are so engrossed in the activity that you lose your self-awareness.[22] It is only afterwards you realize you hadn't been paying a single thought to what had been running through your mind, as if you hadn't been present in that mind for a moment. An activity you can immerse yourself in like that is one of the most blissful things in the world.[23]

You can learn, or lose, the skill to become absorbed in an activity. And people who would like to more often lose themselves in an activity are not helped at all by the world we live in. Materialism, for example, is detrimental to the state of being in which you immerse yourself in something else.[24] And materialism is precisely the attitude and way of thinking drilled into us a thousand times a day, via countless ads that provoke our egos with everything we are apparently lacking. If you want to sleep better, blocking out ads is probably more important than blocking out blue light.

As if sleep itself isn't enough of an incentive, losing yourself in something bigger also comes with an added bonus: enjoyment.

Getting wrapped up in an activity is wonderful. Surrendering yourself is even a prerequisite for any type of enjoyment, Verhaeghe explains. "That point comes up in all classical theories," he says. "Philosophers from Plato to Freud have established that self-awareness and enjoyment do not go together." I think of dancing: I love dancing, but I only actually enjoy it if I'm not busy wondering what I look like, or who is watching me. The less self-conscious I am, the more I enjoy it. An even clearer example is the orgasm: if you are extremely self-aware in bed, it is virtually impossible to reach that climax of enjoyment.

The prerequisite for enjoyment is therefore to get rid of the ego, Verhaeghe says. "Which, incidentally, is also the prerequisite for nodding off." Immerse yourself in something, get wrapped up in something, let yourself be carried away, relax: this is the path to pleasure as well as sleep. Pleasure is associated with relaxation; relaxation is linked to sleep. "It cannot be a coincidence that an orgasmic release is often followed by sleep."

In summary, sleep is not only enjoyable, but you achieve sleep and pleasure via the same route. The key to both is to deactivate your ego.

I think back to my sleep therapist, who urged me to abandon all of my desperate attempts to get some sleep. "The solution to a sleep problem can't be forced. You have to surrender, let go, and let it overcome you. That is something we rarely do in our daily lives anymore."

It wasn't the first time I'd heard something like that, and being constantly told to "let things go" and "simply surrender" infuriated me. Because *how*? Surrender, to what? Let who, or what, overcome you? Morpheus is retired, like all the gods.

But I know how it feels to lose yourself in a wonderful activity, or in a conversation. If there is something you enjoy doing, you don't need to learn to "surrender to something bigger." Simply doing away with your smartphone is a good place to start. And finding companionship. Sleeping works best with someone else, and without too much "me."

After our conversation, Verhaeghe emails me the following formula: "switch off ego + release of stress = pleasure + sleep."

When I read that formula, I think: perhaps insomnia is a blessing after all. A pressing reason to do everything you like doing best. And to connect you more with others. To have more time, to need less money, and to put down roots in the place where you live.

Perhaps the route to sleep actually also leads to happiness.

If happiness and sleep lie in the same direction, justice is also right on that route.

In discussing "others" in relation to sleep I have looked at the damage that a lack of interaction can do, and at the positive effect that fellow humans can have. In the best cases, other people can give you a soporific sense of security. But they can also pose a threat.

This sense of threat is part of why people of color, and women, trans, and gender nonconforming people generally have more problems sleeping. In this book I've mostly written about "men" and "women," since sleep research uses those categories, paying next to no attention to transgender and gender nonconforming people, although preliminary research suggests they frequently have sleep issues. A study among over 200,000 North American college students found they suffered from insomnia and other sleep disorders more often than cisgender students (while also being twice as likely to suffer from depression).[25] Researchers suppose this kind of troubled sleep may be due to the chronic social stress our society imposes on these groups, with hostile treatment leading to increased anxiety, fewer employment options, less job security, and less money, with all the problems that entails.

People of color also face a sleep gap. We've already seen that what you earn, what job you do, what education you've had and where you can afford to live strongly correlate with your chances of a good night's sleep; and that many of those things are unequally distributed between racial groups, with people of color drawing the short straw and noticing the effects of that on their sleep. What 1 haven't discussed is another factor at play in racial sleep disparities, namely: the blunt fact of racism itself. Not operating through wage gaps, substandard housing, or other things, but directly.

Black, Latinx, and Chinese Americans are all much more likely than white people to average less than six hours per night, with Black people going on that little sleep more than double as often as whites.[26] Crucially, if you compare Black and white Americans who are similar in other respects (like income and occupation), the former still sleep less and worse,[27] which is why a number of researchers have posited that the stress of experiencing discrimination plays a role in disrupting sleep.

There is a growing body of research documenting the toll that the experience of discrimination—on grounds of race or ethnicity, and also on the basis of gender, sexuality, or class—takes on physical and mental health. The stress of that experience seems to grind people down; and the fact that it keeps them awake might be at the heart of associated health problems, with depression, anxiety, hypertension, inflammation, cancer, and many others having been linked to the feeling of being discriminated against.[28] It's not only the quantity, but especially the quality of sleep that suffers; people tend to stay more wakeful even during their sleep after an experience of racism, waking more often and having less "deep" sleep.

This is why Tricia Hersey, founder of the Nap Ministry, names sleep deprivation as a racial and social justice issue. Hersey is a performance artist, writer, activist, and theologian, who first started thinking about rest when she was "an exhausted Black woman in America living in the South, going to an all-white institution."[29] Already holding a bachelor's degree in public health, she was aware of the vital importance of sleep, and the fact that people of color were getting less of it. As she was conducting research into Black plantation labor, she started to connect Black people's current relationship with sleep and rest to this history of oppression.

She notices many Black people feel they have to overachieve to prove their worth; the idea of the Black "superwoman," for instance, comes at the cost of sleep.[30] This is partly in response to the racist stereotype of Black people as inherently "lazy," "a stereotype that justified whipping as the antidote to exhaustion on plantations and is still weaponized today."[31] Capitalism values productivity over the natural need to rest, and slavery was capitalism's first experiment: to work a human being like a machine.[32] Hersey summarizes capitalism's message as: "Your body doesn't belong to you, keep working, you are simply a tool for our production."[33]

If you do not take time to rest, you are aligning yourself with that system, and being violent towards your own body. "When you don't sleep, you're literally killing your body. It's not a dramatic over-the-top thing to say that." The same machine-level pace of labor that was used on the plantation "drives capitalism and grind culture today."[34] This culture tries to convince us we are worthless unless we are busy producing, consuming, creating. "You have to see that grind culture is violent, it's an extension of white supremacy, it doesn't look at you as a human being."[35]

Therefore she urges Black people especially to embrace rest as a form of resistance; to detox from technology and take some time to rest and daydream every day, even if it's just ten minutes. Her Nap Ministry's signature events are Collective Napping Experiences, harnessing the power of coming together as a community for healing.[36]

As Nap Bishop, Hersey is spreading the gospel of sleep and rest, stressing also its spiritual powers: its way of opening a space for imagination, a dream space, a portal for ideas. For her, rest holds a spiritual message in its unspoken claim that human beings have the right to just be; that they do not have to prove their worth by toiling to exhaustion, because they are already divine.[37]

In short, a nap is "more than a nap: it's pushback and disruption," Hersey says.[38] To rest is to push back and say: "My body doesn't belong to capitalism. My body belongs to me."[39]

00:00
THE WEIGHT
OF SLEEP

WHEN I LIE AWAKE in the middle of the night in a state of hyperarousal, I often feel like I am floating. Perhaps the involuntary muscle tension is the reason why I'm not sinking into the mattress, but lying on top of it. Regardless, it feels like I am weightless, a helium balloon caught between the sheets. My thoughts pull me in all directions, and the weight of my body is barely enough to keep me in my place.

Sleeplessness is weightlessness.

The same thing came to mind when I read the diaries of Kafka—another writer who was an insomniac. I was looking for references to his nights, hoping to recognize myself in him or to understand how he dealt with his insomnia. In doing so I stumbled upon a passage in which he describes the position he assumed in bed at night: his arms crossed over his chest with his hands on his shoulders "like a heavily laden soldier." He tries to make himself as heavy as possible, he writes, as weight helps when it comes to sleep. It was a touching image: the serious Kafka lying in that funny position on his back, waiting for sleep.

But what if his intuition that we need weight to fall asleep was right? I thought about my boyfriend, who would come and squash me on my request. And about the weighted blanket I had been sent. About the calm voice in my head-phones trying to convince me that my legs were getting heavy.

Sometimes it helped a bit. But usually not enough.

Two households of furniture were packed into the van my boyfriend and I hired for our house move. The loading space was filled to the roof, the passenger space was full of people and their luggage. Because we had loaded the van so full, it lowed like a pregnant cow. On the highway it barely reached thirty miles an hour going uphill.

When we had almost arrived at our destination, it looked like we weren't going to make the final, steep turn. We were stranded in the pitch-dark night, on the corner of the road we were moving to. In the light of our headlights and our mobile phones, we got out to push. With squealing tires, it conquered the final ascent.

The next morning the friends who had traveled with us helped unload everything. Then they drove the same van back again, which was now high on its wheels. We watched as it bounced off jauntily down the road. My boyfriend and I kept waving, tears in our eyes, until it was out of sight. Afterwards, we looked at each other in shock.

All of the weight had been left with us.

At the time of writing the last chapter of this book, a year has passed and that weight has further increased. My life doesn't have much in common with the one of the unat-tached, insomniac urban dweller who started researching insomnia—a project that put more in motion than I could have anticipated.

If I wanted to move house again now, that van definitely wouldn't suffice. Even if only because of Kepler, the black border collie with a galaxy of spots on his white snout. When he came to live with us, he weighed four pounds and was so nervous he peed on my lap. Now he weighs forty and runs around on his own through the village, which he thinks he owns. He has his regular haunts; he knows exactly which neighbor saves bones for him after lunch, where he can roll around in fresh cow manure, and when the neighbor cleans out her guinea pig hutch, so he can sniff around in the straw.

As Kepler grew, I got bigger too. With a bulging tummy, I did jobs around the house and worked in the garden. Neighbors reprimanded me when they saw me ("Do I need to remind you that you are pregnant?"). I shovelled four tons of compost into wheelbarrows, lugged twenty rolls of glass wool into the attic.

My subletter from then now sleeps in her own bed, and weighs so much that the pediatrician asks, "Are you giving her fertilizer?"

For a long time I thought I needed to be more light-footed, more light-hearted, in order to sleep. Unencumbered. I dreamed of emptiness, of absolute nothingness.

In bed I imagined that everything would suddenly reset to zero when my alarm jumped from 23:59 to midnight. No thoughts anymore, no inner unrest; my mind an uncreased, starched bedsheet. Or I imagined that the clock would stay on one minute to twelve for just as long as it took me to fall asleep. Instead, after the magical string of zeros, it simply started counting again from scratch.

The "reset" I lusted after didn't come about by magic, or at midnight. In order to achieve that, I had to emigrate, in a van that slogged its way up the Burgundian hills.

I didn't sleep very well that first night in our ice-cold house. The second night I slept deeply; it was already light when I woke up. I stared incredulously at the alarm clock. I had slept for almost ten hours in a row.

A stroke of luck? An exception? Perhaps, but the exception continued.

After a week, my boyfriend, also a bad sleeper, joked about this strange new situation in which we would lie down in bed and simply fall asleep. "Perhaps we should run a sleep course," he said. "Step one: pack up your entire home. Step two: ensure your bedroom temperature is just above freezing."

At first we thought it might have been due to the exhaustion of the move. And later, due to the physical exertion of renovating, hauling, unpacking, painting. But it continued, even when we returned to our laptops. Despite the puppy that had to be let out twice a night the first few months; despite the stress of COVID-19, despite breaking every sleep hygiene rule in the book; despite the physical discomforts of pregnancy and despite the baby who now regularly summons me for night feeds, my sleep is still incomparably better than I remember it being at any other point in my adult life. A change I wouldn't have been so sure of if it hadn't come about so abruptly and gone on for so long.

Admittedly, this is what I had hoped for when I turned my life upside down. That hope had been an important reason for taking the leap. But I hadn't really expected it.

If I lie awake at night these days, I can almost always think of a reason why. A hornet is buzzing around in our bedroom;

I am mulling over a tricky phrase in a text; Kepler has eaten a mothball and I am worried. The pointless, incomprehensible tossing and turning that once drove me to despair is now a thing of the past.

Incidentally, I am not the first person to turn my life around in the hope of being able to get some sleep. The American writer Henry David Thoreau, for example, preceded me. His insomnia was so severe that it reduced him to "a diseased bundle of nerves," as he wrote in his diary. It left him barely able to read or write. He retreated to a secluded hut for two years in the hope he would finally be able to sleep, and the result was sleep *and* the book *Walden*.[1]

Reflecting on my voyage to sleep, I keep coming back to the term "weight."

In high school I learned that weight, in scientific terms, is the force exerted by gravity on an object. I can no longer recall the details, but I can see the picture in front of me that accompanied the explanation in the textbook. It was an image of a wheelbarrow piled high with wood. In the middle of the pile was a red dot, from which an arrow pointed straight down to the ground, so that it looked like what was in the wheelbarrow was putting down roots. The greater the weight, the deeper the roots and the more difficult it was to move the wheelbarrow. Weight was a force that kept things in place.

That wasn't something that appealed to me. I didn't want to stay in place; I was ambitious. I wanted to grow in all directions like a tree stretching its branches here, there, and everywhere. I didn't stop to think that a tree had to stretch just as far in the dark under the ground as in the sky above it. If the root system isn't as extensive as the canopy, it can easily fall down.

Let's return to the image of a wheelbarrow with weight shooting down to the ground from it like a root. "Weight" offers a connecting thread that links together the building blocks I just mentioned: money, time, place, and others.

Let's take the connection between time and money. I already described how I have more time left over since I started living with less money. Whenever I make a trade-off between the two, I try to choose time. Of the two supposedly convertible entities, *time* is best at exerting a force that keeps you in your place. Contrary to money, it is a fundamental element of every human experience; you can't experience anything outside of time. And that's why time weighs considerably more than money.

Imagine you want to get to the top of a mountain. You could take a cable car, but that costs money. Or you could walk there, but that takes time. In the hours you spend walking, you notice the flowers alongside the path getting smaller as you get higher; the physical exertion causes the blood to whoosh in your ears; the view gradually opens up until you reach the top, from where you can take in the whole panorama. It is clear which of the two options will leave a more lasting impression.

Another example could be a gift that you make yourself instead of buying. Buying means a financial sacrifice, and that can be meaningful, depending on the size of your wallet. You are also giving some of your time indirectly, because you have probably earned that money by working. But if you make something yourself you are spending that time directly, and everything is included in those hours: evidence of your (lack of) dexterity, your personal tastes, and the impression you have of the recipient, but above all, the fact that you were probably constantly thinking of them as you were making it. That can sometimes make a homemade gift almost too charged with meaning. There are just a handful of people, only very good friends, to whom I would feel comfortable giving a homemade gift. It can soon feel like too much.

So, more time, and less money. That also means: slower days, with more space between the "cookie dough" (and more time to actually bake something). The hours aren't as crammed full, but at the same time, they are fuller. They seem to have a different texture, they are more sensually dense, as if someone has fiddled with the filters: the color saturation and the richness of sound have been intensified. Perhaps this impression of saturation simply occurs because I am less tired and able to take more in. Or because I have the time to look more closely. Either way, the days are denser. They feel sturdier now that they can take root in the night.

And then there's the weight of others. That used to attract me but also put me off: I was afraid that a potential relationship would go wrong or that I wouldn't be able to cope with the responsibility of a dog, for example, and certainly not a child. Now they seem to help root me: the weight of the man to whom I bound myself by emigrating; that of the dog who enjoys putting his paws on my keyboard while I work; and that of the infant who is now so heavy that I've developed tendonitis in my wrists.

Then there are the other villagers. There was a time when I would have been annoyed if a neighbor had come to sit on my sofa and burst out in tears because of some personal drama or other. I would have thought: I don't have the time for this. But now I love the fact she feels comfortable to do that and that her little boy comes to get us because he wants to show off his new treehouse.

Another reason why I feel so at home here is because of a third type of weight: the support my environment offers. The house, the garden, the village, and the surrounding woods play an important role in my daily life. According to my dictionary, gravity is the "Earth's pull," and I can clearly sense that here.

As a writer, my work involves my thoughts being elsewhere; I spend a great deal of time daydreaming. One of the best changes is therefore a sturdier "here"; a place that invites you to linger. Here I can walk into the garden and simply pull vegetables out of the ground for dinner. Here the weather forecast determines when I put the washing on. Here warmth can be carried inside, in the form of arms full of wood from the shed. Here in spring we first conquer the sunny pavement in front of the house, then the garden, then the whole valley; in the dead of winter only the few feet around the stove are really comfortable. In this way our environment expands and then shrinks again over the course of the year, as if we are living with the slow breathing of a gigantic being.

Although I hadn't felt that anything was missing from my life in the city, I now realize that I was lacking the weight of an environment that had something concrete and solid for me. I no longer need to do exercises in the evening to feel my body getting heavy, because that strong sense of being physically present in a certain place remains with me at night. I am like my dog who, stretched out on the rug, keeps running through the fields in his sleep: his speckled paws move in the rhythm of a trot.

The weight I was once so suspicious of now presents itself in accordance with its official definition: as a force. Weight, I think now, also means sturdiness, importance. Without weight, even the smallest breeze can blow you over.

My personal experiences are not a magic formula, but are intended to serve as an illustration. My intention is simply to open up a new avenue to explore in a situation in which it may feel like there is no way out: chronic insomnia.

It may seem strange to seek solutions on such a large scale. "Take a close, critical look at your life" is not advice you come across in the usual popular scientific articles about sleep, or in the never-ending lists of tips for a better night's sleep.

The Harvard Medical School, for example, an institute that represents the latest scientific knowledge, concludes an article about sleeplessness with a list of tips aimed at combatting your insomnia. These tips include: move more, do relaxation exercises, improve your sleep hygiene (no TV in your bedroom, etc.), and limit alcohol and coffee. This falls under the heading "lifestyle changes."[2]

As far as I am aware, the idea that changing the *style* of your life is perhaps not enough, and that instead, you need to take a look at the very *core* of it, never appears on such lists.[3]

These lists are incomplete. They only focus on one of the three causes of sleeping problems: physical factors (such as sleep hygiene, the amount of caffeine you drink, or your genetic predisposition to hyperarousal). They might, on occasion, dedicate a couple of sentences to the second type: psychological factors, such as the pressure you feel to fall asleep quickly at night. But the third category is almost always ignored: contextual factors, such as time pressure, income, living environment, and loneliness.

I do not wish to deny the role of physical factors in insomnia, but instead intend to supplement it with something I consider essential, based on my own experience. I had already worked my way through the first two categories. I had followed all the practical sleep tips and insofar as the psychological category was concerned, I had sought therapy more than once. It was never enough. I thought to myself: this is hopeless. I *am* an insomniac. It's all part and parcel of who I am.

I see it differently now. Not because I underestimate the role of physical or psychological factors, and not because I deny that I am susceptible to insomnia in these fields. (I have noticed, for example, that I still struggle with sleep if I am under a lot of pressure, like in the exhausting weeks after giving birth; when I finally had the opportunity to lie down during the day, I simply couldn't sleep.)

I expect that sleep will always be a delicate issue for me, however I arrange my life. But what I am better able to recognize now is that a sensitivity doesn't have to be painful. You need an irritant for that. And that might be found in the way you are living.

A susceptibility to insomnia can be something useful too. Canaries didn't get taken down the coal mines because they flourished there, but because they were sensitive to the poisonous gases that would otherwise go unnoticed. Sleep, my own personal canary, hangs its head if I feel lonely, sense a great pressure to "ego-build" or suffer from financial stresses and the associated time pressures, or find myself in a living environment that isn't very meaningful to me.

Your list may be different, but the principle remains the same: you can use your insomnia as a call to action. That's why I would love to supplement all the lists of sleeping tips. "If lifestyle tips don't work, don't change your lifestyle. Change your life."

I recently tried to describe this book to an acquaintance from our village: the local forester, a man of few words. He listened to my account of the connection between sleep, loneliness, money, time pressure, and a lack of rootedness, went silent for a moment, and then summarized: "So, you need to be happy in order to sleep."

I was taken aback for a moment. Had I needed a whole *book* for that? But then I thought: yes, that is a good conclusion. If insomnia encourages you to take steps in a direction that makes you happier, the extra sleep you might collect en route is perhaps the smaller win.

I can imagine that the extensive suggestions in this book might seem intimidating. Especially if you are very tired. You might be thinking that nobody is able to really change the things I have written about *on their own*. But if you want to get to the root of the sleep problems so prevalent in today's society, you need to look beyond self-help. Financial insecurity, time pressure, a lack of rootedness, and loneliness are topics that are so vast, so omnipresent, and so intertwined with the way in which today's world functions that you can only *really* change them by political means. Ultimately, the question of sleep asks: In what kind of world do we want to live? In what kind of world would we be able to sleep again?

It might be frustrating to read a self-help book whose conclusions you are unable to fully implement. The things that
keep us up are often bigger than us, and we are caught up in
the middle of them. But this entanglement also contains a
solution. Insomnia can feel very lonely, but there are plenty
of others listening to the same warning signal who also
want to do something about it. This common desire could
trigger a collective change, which could have consequences
that extend way beyond sleep.

If I am ever unable to sleep these days, *that's* where my
thoughts take me. Instead of obsessing over which sleep
hygiene rule I might have broken, I wonder whether my
lack of sleep might be saying something about the bigger
picture—my life, my environment, and the role I am playing
or would like to be playing in it. It seems sensible to ponder
that for a while.

Through the skylight above me I see part of the sky, full
of stars. If I look for long enough, they move in relation to
the window frame, witnesses to the slow revolution I am
making down below. On a clear night, from my pillow I can
even see the Milky Way.

ACKNOWLEDGEMENTS

A NUMBER OF FRAGMENTS included in this book have already been published in a different format.

A column about the IKEA effect was published in *Psychologie Magazine* (September 2020).

The series "Hoe slaapt de 21e eeuw?" (How does the 21st century sleep?), from which I have incorporated parts in this book in a very modified form, appeared in *Vrij Nederland*. This series came about with support from the Dutch Fund for In-Depth Journalism.

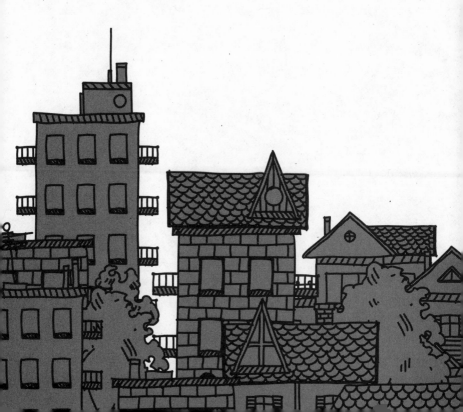

NOTES

01:00
All Animals Sleep

1 For the sleeping behavior of elephant seals, see: Yoko Mitani et al., "Three-Dimensional Resting Behaviour of Northern Elephant Seals: Drifting Like a Falling Leaf," *Biology Letters*, Vol. 6, No. 2 (2010), pp. 163–166.

2 See: Matthew Walker, *Why We Sleep: Unlocking the Power of Sleep and Dreams* (New York: Penguin, 2018).

3 Based on figures from 2017, Statistics Netherlands reveals that one in five Dutch people aged twelve and up report sleep problems. One in ten report many or very many sleep problems. See: Statistics Netherlands "Een op de vijf meldt slaapproblemen" (16 March 2018).

4 Half is an approximation. According to research carried out by TeamAlert in 2019, 42.7 percent of young people don't sleep long enough,

43.4 percent feel they sleep badly, and as many as 65.2 percent actually sleep badly according to the researchers' criteria. See: TeamAlert, "Onderzoek Jongeren en Slapen," 2019. Other research reveals that there are big differences between how adolescent boys and girls sleep: while 31.3 percent of boys suffer from sleep disturbance (such as waking often or too early and struggling to fall asleep), such disturbance applies to 52.7 percent of girls. See: Gerard Kerkhof, "Epidemiology of Sleep and Sleep Disorders in the Netherlands," *Sleep Medicine*, Vol. 30 (2017), pp. 229–239.

5 Namely: they sleep badly and do not get enough sleep, have trouble initiating or maintaining sleep, and the sleep disturbance significantly impacts their day-to-day life.

And their complaints persist: for at least three nights per week, for at least three months in a row. Furthermore, the sleep disturbance is not attributable to too much coffee, a painful illness, or depression, for example. If that is the case, it does not count as insomnia. These are the criteria according to the DSM-5, the *Diagnostic and Statistical Manual of Mental Disorders*, 5th edition. The one in ten figure is when you measure at any one point in time; if you look at people sleeping this badly throughout a given year, the figures are even higher. Approximately 30 percent to 40 percent of adults in the United States report symptoms of insomnia at some point in a given year. See: Julie A. Dopheide, "Insomnia Overview: Epidemiology, Pathophysiology, Diagnosis and Monitoring, and Nonpharmacologic Therapy," *American Journal of Managed Care* (April 2020).

6   As far as we know, other animals do not experience insomnia the same way humans do. By this I mean *attempting* to sleep and failing even though you have the opportunity to do so. All sorts of research has been carried out on animals that stay awake more than usual, but they are usually intentionally *kept*

awake by the researchers. If, for example, you put rats in a wheel that never stops turning, they won't be able to sleep; but it is difficult to compare this situation with one of a person lying awake in a safe, quiet bedroom, "in the calmest and most stillest night, / with all appliances and means to boot" (Shakespeare). It also seems that animals that don't get much movement and are kept in captivity—such as horses in a stable—stay awake for an unusually long time at night. However, as far as I know, insomnia has not been observed among animals in the wild (in their normal habitat). This raises the question whether humans are not, in some way, living in captivity. See: Linda Toth and Pavan Bhargava, "Animal Models of Sleep Disorders," *Comparative Medicine*, Vol. 63, No. 2 (2013), pp. 91–104. For the awake horses, see: "Do Animals Have Sleep Disorders?," Sleepandhealth.com, an article that is probably based on Christine Fuchs, "Narkolepsie oder REM-Schlafmangel? 24-Stunden-Überwachung und polysomnographische Messungen bei adulten 'narkoleptischen' Pferden," dissertation, LMU München (2017).

02:00
Sleep as a
Waste of Time

1 David Gelles et al., "Elon Musk Details 'Excruciating' Personal Toll of Tesla Turmoil," *New York Times* (16 August 2016).

2 Alan Derickson, *Dangerously Sleepy: Overworked Americans and the Cult of Manly Wakefulness* (Philadelphia: University of Pennsylvania Press, 2014).

3 Researchers often look at modern hunter-gatherers, under the assumption that they follow an "archetypal pattern" in one way or another, but that's questionable; the few groups that still depend on hunting and gathering are each faced with specific circumstances and each have their own culture: factors that influence the way they sleep. In general, these hunter-gatherers don't appear to sleep especially long, for example between 6.45 and 8.15 hours depending on the season. Other researchers sift through old diaries, letters, or criminal documents, looking for references to sleep, and try to put the pieces of the puzzle together with these snippets of information. As such, it seems that people from Antwerp in the eighteenth century slept about seven hours per night, already falling short of the gold standard of eight hours. The wealthier residents of Antwerp were an exception, often being able to stay in bed much longer than the plebs. See: Gerrit Verhoeven, "(Pre)Modern Sleep: New Evidence From the Antwerp Criminal Court (1715-1795)," *Journal of Sleep Research*, Wiley Online Library (11 June 2020). Considering there weren't any painkillers, the beds were swarming with vermin, and many people shared their homes with all sorts of livestock, this sub-ideal sleep is not especially surprising.

4 Plato, for example, dictated that citizens should sleep less than slaves, as sleep is "dead time" for those with things to do. Shakespeare's Henry IV envies his "poorest subjects" for their ability to sleep soundly at night, because despite his more comfortable bed, he is weighed down by his responsibilities: "Uneasy lies the head that wears a crown." See: Kimberley Whitehead and Matthew Beaumont, "Insomnia: A Brief Cultural History," *Lancet*, Vol. 391, No. 10138 (2016), pp. 2408-2409.

5 For the changing view on sleep, see: A. Roger Ekirch,

At Day's Close: Night in Times Past (New York: W.W. Norton, 2005).

6   The contemporary version of this view is articulated impressively by Jonathan Crary. In his book, *24/7: Late Capitalism and the Ends of Sleep* (New York: Verso, 2013), he outlines how capitalism penetrates every aspect of our lives. Crary claims that sleep, the time when people are not productive and not actively consuming, is an enemy of capitalism. He portrays sleep as an act of resistance against a world in which importance is only measured in dollars. Georges Perec offers a literary counterpart to this in *A Man Asleep*. In this novella, a Parisian student opts out of "this enveloping atmosphere of obligations, this eternal machine for producing, crushing, swallowing up," and decides instead to sleep. See: Georges Perec, *A Man Asleep*, translated by Andrew Leak (New York: Vintage, 2011).

7   Derickson, *Dangerously Sleepy*, chapter 1.

8   Ibid. The claim of "two hours" is taken from Laird's *Increasing Personal Efficiency* (New York: Harper, 1925).

9   See the World Health Organization report, "WHO Technical Meeting on Sleep and Health," 2004.

10 See: Kerkhof, "Epidemiology of Sleep and Sleep Disorders in the Netherlands." See also: Statistics Netherlands: "Een op de vijf meldt slaapproblemen" (16 March 2018).

11 According to the Gallup poll, in 1942, just 36 percent slept seven hours or less, and 11 percent averaged six hours or less. See: Jeffrey M. Jones, "In U.S., 40 Percent Get Less Than Recommended Amount of Sleep," Gallup (19 December 2013). The U.S. Centers for Disease Control and Prevention reported in 2014 that just over 35 percent of Americans sleep more than seven hours per night.

12 According to the Royal Society for Public Health, 2016. See: Haroon Siddique, "Britons Missing an Hour's Sleep Every Night, Says Report," *The Guardian* (1 April 2016).

13 According to a poll among a representative sample of the population by the insurance company Aviva, 2018. "U.K. Adults Missing Out on 11 Hours of Sleep Each Week."

14 Darian Leader, *Why Can't We Sleep? Understanding Our Sleeping and Sleepless Minds* (New York: Penguin, 2019). A nap (*wu shuy*) was usually taken during the lunchtime rest, or *xiu xi*, which was specifically included in Mao's constitution. See: Leo Benedictus, "The Art of the Urban Nap: Let's Lose the Stigma of Public Snoozing," *The Guardian* (7 July 2015).

15 I have been unable to substantiate Walker's claim; there are also sources that contradict him. It is possible that coffee was temporarily the second-most-traded commodity in the world—in the 1970s—but MIT's *Observatory of Economic Complexity* currently ranks coffee at number 98.

16 "The consumption of caffeine represents one of the longest and largest unsupervised drug studies ever conducted on the human race, perhaps rivaled only by alcohol, and it continues to this day." See: Walker, *Why We Sleep*, chapter 2.

03:00
Sleep as Performance

1 In the Netherlands, with a blood alcohol content of 0.05 percent, you are no longer permitted to drive. If you are caught with a blood alcohol content of 0.08 percent, you are required to attend a driver improvement course. This example is taken from Walker, *Why We Sleep*.

2 In the United States alone, thirty additional deaths, and $175 million of costs are attributed to this each year. See: Austin C. Smith, "Spring Forward at Your Own Risk: Daylight Saving Time and Fatal Vehicle Crashes," *American Economic Journal: Applied Economics*, Vol. 8, No. 2 (2016), pp. 65–91.

3 Approximately half of the 196 CEOs who responded to an international survey wrongly believed that lack of sleep didn't affect their functioning. See: Nick van Dam and Els van der Helm, "The Organizational Cost of Insufficient Sleep," *McKinsey Quarterly* (February 2016).

4 There is an identifiable hormonal cause of your increased appetite. Lack of sleep causes the concentration of the hormone that signals

to your brain that you are full (leptin) to decrease, whereas the concentration of the "give me more" hormone (ghrelin) increases. That's why people who don't get enough sleep have bigger appetites and less self-control. Interview with Els van der Helm (5 March 2019).

5   Christopher M. Barnes, "Research: Your Abusive Boss Is Probably an Insomniac," *Harvard Business Review* (7 November 2014).

6   I spoke to Dr. Robbert Havekes, researcher at the University of Groningen, about this. Interview with Robbert Havekes (11 March 2019).

7   See: Scott Davis et al., "Night Shift Work, Light at Night, and Risk of Breast Cancer," *JNCI: Journal of the National Cancer Institute*, Vol. 93, No. 20 (17 October 2001), pp. 1557–1562. In chapter 8 of his book, Walker (*Why We Sleep*, 2018) writes that sleeping six hours or less is associated with a 40 percent increased risk of developing cancer, relative to those sleeping seven hours a night or more. The exact percentages depend on the type of cancer.

8   Shankar Vedantam, "The Haunting Effects of Going Days Without Sleep," *NPR*

(27 December 2017). See also Walker, *Why We Sleep*, chapter 4.

9   Van der Helm (who admittedly stands to benefit from an overestimation in view of the product she is selling) estimates that lack of sleep for an imaginary employee with a gross salary of 70,000 euros per year equates to an annual loss of productivity equivalent to 15,000 euros. An estimate published in the *Journal of Occupational and Environmental Medicine* in January 2010 identifies an average productivity loss of $1,967 per employee per year. See: Mark Rosekind et al., "The Cost of Poor Sleep: Workplace Productivity Loss and Associated Costs," *Journal of Occupational and Environmental Medicine*, Vol. 52, No. 1 (January 2010), pp. 91–98. The research company RAND calculated that lack of sleep, in the form of decreased productivity and increased healthcare costs, can reduce gross domestic product by up to 3 percent. That's more than many countries spend on defense. If the shortest sleepers—those who get six hours or less—would sleep an hour longer, it would generate billions for a country. See: Marco Hafner et al., "Why Sleep Matters—the Economic Costs of Insufficient

Sleep: A Cross-Country Comparative Analysis," *RAND Corporation* (2016).

10 See: Carol Connolly et al., "Sleep Well, Lead Well: How Better Sleep Can Improve Leadership, Boost Productivity, and Spark Innovation," Center for Creative Leadership (2014), p. 8.

11 This slogan is attributed to the Belgian surrealist Louis Scutenaire. See: "Louis Scutenaire, le provocateur," *Le Monde* (23 July 1982).

12 Darian Leader, "Why the Sleep Industry Is Keeping Us Awake at Night," *The Guardian* (13 March 2019).

13 Alan Ohnsman, "Elon Musk May Not Be Working All the Hours He Claims, but Boy He Needs Sleep," *Forbes* (17 August 2018).

04:00
In Search of Sleep

1 This is the "group edge effect." See: Niels Rattenborg et al., "Half-Awake to the Risk of Predation," *Nature*, Vol. 397, No. 6718 (1999), pp. 397–398. It should be noted that this does not apply during REM sleep: all birds sleep with both halves of the brain during that phase. See: Walker, *Why We Sleep*, chapter 4.

05:00
Sleeping Pills
Don't Work

1 These numbers are limited to benzodiazepines like oxazepam and temazepam, and don't include other types of sleeping pill like zopiclone. See: Stichting Farmaceutische Kengetallen, "Gebruik benzodiazepines vorig jaar verder afgenomen," *Pharmaceutisch Weekblad*, Vol. 153, No. 3 (18 January 2018).

2 In research among 86,000 adults, 12.6 percent of people reported having used benzodiazepines in the past year. Donovan T. Maust et al., "Benzodiazepine Use and Misuse Among Adults in the United States," *Psychiatric Services*, Vol. 70, No. 2 (2 February 2019), pp. 97–106. These figures don't even take into account other medical sleep aids like Z-drugs or SSRIs. For the monthly prescription rates of all of these, see S.A. Milani et al., "Trends in the Use of Benzodiazepines, Z-Hypnotics, and Serotonergic Drugs Among U.S. Women and Men Before and During the COVID-19 Pandemic," *JAMA Network Open*, Vol. 4, No. 10 (25 October 2021).

3   Ibid. Those aged eighteen to twenty-four use as many benzodiazepines with prescription as without, the latter being termed misuse. For the same group, sleep aid prescriptions tripled between 1998 and 2006, according to a market research firm. Julie Steenhuysen, "Use of Sleep Aids by Young U.S. Adults Soars: Study," Reuters (16 January 2009).

4   Canadian Drug Summary: Sedatives, May 2022, Canadian Centre on Substance Use and Addiction. In Canada, 11.2 percent of drivers killed in vehicle accidents between 2000 and 2010 tested positive for sedative-hypnotic prescription drugs post-mortem. See: J. Brandt and C. Leong, "Benzodiazepines and Z-Drugs: An Updated Review of Major Adverse Outcomes Reported on in Epidemiologic Research," *Drugs in R&D*, Vol. 17, No. 4 (December 2017), pp. 493–507.

5   For instance, a small study among 1,500 people in the U.K. found that more than a quarter of people between sixteen and fifty-nine had taken benzodiazepines or Z-drugs at some point; and almost 8 percent of adults had taken them without prescription. V. Kapil et al., "Misuse of Benzodiazepines and Z-Drugs in the U.K.," *British Journal of Psychiatry*, Vol. 205, No. 5 (2 January 2018), pp. 407–408.

6   This and the following quotations: interview with Eus van Someren (20 February 2019).

7   The researchers state that the effect of sleeping pills is "rather small and of questionable clinical importance." It concerned pills such as zopiclone and zolpidem. See: Tania Huedo-Medina et al., "Effectiveness of Non-Benzodiazepine Hypnotics in Treatment of Adult Insomnia: Meta-Analysis of Data Submitted to the Food and Drug Administration," *British Medical Journal*, Vol. 345 (2012).

8   A meta-analysis carried out by Harvard Medical School, which compared twenty different studies into the effect of cognitive behavioral therapy on sleeping problems, concluded that this type of therapy results in someone falling asleep twenty minutes sooner and being awake for half an hour less during the night, on average. Furthermore, this effect continued after the end of the therapy. James Trauer et al., "Cognitive Behavioral Therapy of Chronic Insomnia: A Systematic Review and Meta-Analysis,"

Annals of Internal Medicine, Vol. 163, No. 3 (4 August 2015). "These improvements are as good as, or better than, those seen in people who take prescription sleep medications such as zolpidem (Ambien) and eszopiclone (Lunesta). And unlike medications, the effects of CBT-I last even after the therapy ends—at least six months, according to one study," Harvard summarizes. See: Julie Corliss, "Cognitive Behavioral Therapy Offers a Drug-Free Method for Managing Insomnia," *Harvard Health Blog* (10 June 2015).

9   A major study of 10,000 users of sleeping pills revealed that they were almost five times as likely to die during the two-and-a-half-year duration of the study than those who didn't take sleeping pills. Users of sleeping pills appeared to have a significantly greater risk of developing cancer during those two and a half years than the control group. The more pills, the greater the likelihood, but even those who took between one and eighteen pills per year were more likely to develop cancer. See: Daniel Kripke et al., "Hypnotics' Association With Mortality or Cancer: A Matched Cohort Study," *BMJ Open* (27 February 2012). Walker

(*Why We Sleep*, 2018) suggests an increase of 40 to 60 percent on the basis of this and other studies. Walker explains that it is possible that the cancer was caused by something other than sleeping pills—for example, the users of sleeping pills not getting any "proper" sleep, so being less able to benefit from the restorative effects of sleep. However, that would still hardly be an ad for sleeping pills. A study of 15,000 Taiwanese people revealed that those who took Ambien were 68 percent more likely to get cancer. See: C.-H. Kao et al., (2012). "Relationship of Zolpidem and Cancer Risk: A Taiwanese Population-Based Cohort Study," *Mayo Clinic Proceedings*, Vol. 87, No. 5 (2012), pp. 430–436.

06:00
Desperately Trying to Relax

1   What follows is a simplified, condensed rendering of various sessions and a telephone interview a few months afterwards.

2   Telephone interview with Sanne Verkooijen (3 April 2019).

07:00
We Don't Know
a Lot About Sleep

1 Another term for this is "paradoxical insomnia." The paradox is that the insomniac suffers from insomnia, but that it doesn't actually exist, at least according to the EEG.

08:00
Sleep Isn't Black
and White

1 A loss of muscle tension is another characteristic of REM sleep, and together with eye movement activity serves as an additional criterion to determine whether someone is actually in this phase of sleep. See Walker, *Why We Sleep*, chapter 3.

2 You wake up more easily during NREM 1 than during NREM 3, for example. However, that is not the only difference. People in NREM 1 most often have involuntary muscle twitches, and people in the deepest and last phase of NREM are most likely to display "parasomnias": striking behaviors such as sleepwalking, eating, talking, or even having sex in their sleep. Matthew Walker and Darian Leader both write clearly about these phases of sleep.

3 Walker, *Why We Sleep*, chapter 9.

4 Today, NREM is usually divided into three phases, of which NREM 3 is the deepest. That is the phase in which bad nightmares occur. The fact that you can't usually remember the dreams or nightmares you had during NREM sleep the next day does not mean that you didn't have any. It could even be the case that you deliberately forget them, and that NREM evades your memory because it has more to hide. See: Leader (2019).

5 Adrian Owen et al., "Detecting Awareness in the Vegetative State," *Science*, Vol. 313, No. 5792 (2016), p. 1402.

6 Adrian Owen, "How Science Found a Way to Help Coma Patients Communicate," *The Guardian* (5 September 2017).

7 Interview with Eus van Someren (20 February 2019).

8 The European Road Safety Observatory states in a 2021 report that 15 to 20 percent of serious crashes are caused by fatigue, and refers to a large-scale international survey showing that between 20 and 25 percent of the car drivers indicated that, during the last month, they had driven at least once while they were so sleepy that they had

trouble keeping their eyes open. According to SWOV Institute for Road Safety Research, fatigue is the cause of 15 to 20 percent of all road traffic collisions. See: "Fatigue Factsheet," SWOV (September 2019). In chapter 19 of *Why We Sleep*, Walker writes that a lack of sleep is more lethal than drugs and alcohol *put together*, but I have been unable to verify this claim. Statistics from the United States suggest that approximately 21 percent of fatal road traffic collisions can be attributed to sleep deprivation, compared to 28 percent to drunk driving. See respectively: "Drowsy Driving Is Impaired Driving," National Security Council (2017), and "Impaired Driving Factsheet," Centers for Disease Control and Prevention (24 August 2020).

9   Masako Tamaki et al., "Night Watch in One Brain Hemisphere Associated With the First-Night Effect in Humans," *Current Biology*, Vol. 26, No. 9 (9 May 2016), pp. 1190–1194.

10:00
Hyperarousal

1   Interview with Sanne Verkooijen (3 April 2019).

2   The official term for that system is the "sympathetic nervous system"; it triggers the fight-or-flight response.

11:00
The Bright Side of Hyperarousal

1   As lots of studies lump these two groups together, it is virtually impossible for me not to do the same. Where possible, I have differentiated between a "lack of sleep" and "sleep problems" in this book, whereby the former relates to good sleepers who aren't getting enough sleep and the latter relates to problematic sleepers, including those with an official diagnosis of insomnia.

2   Sleep problems are not limited to insomnia: sleep apnea, periodic limb movement disorder, narcolepsy, and so on are all classed as "sleep problems." I will use the term mainly with regard to difficulty falling asleep and staying asleep.

3   Vladimir Nabokov, *Speak, Memory* (New York: Penguin, 2000 [1951]).

4   The American poet Dana Gioia also refers to this in his poem "Insomnia": "The terrible clarity this moment brings, / the useless insight, the unbroken dark." For Cioran, see Willis G. Regier, "Cioran's Insomnia," *MLN*, Vol. 119, No. 5, Comparative Literature Issue (December 2004), pp. 994–1012.

5   Gabriel Liiceanu, *Itinéraires d'une vie: E. M. Cioran* (Paris: Michalon, 1990), p. 92. My translation.

6   "The importance of insomnia is so colossal that I am tempted to define man as the animal who cannot sleep. Why call him a rational animal when other animals are equally reasonable? But there is not another animal in the entire creation that wants to sleep yet cannot." Cioran, *On the Heights of Despair*, translated by Ilinca Zarifopol-Johnston (Chicago: Chicago University Press, 1992), p. 58.

7   And singers, such as the unnamed Inuit singers of "Utitia'q's Song," who sing about a man who got lost on the ice. The last verse of this song expresses the lucidity that follows a long period without sleep in a wonderfully simple manner: "When I tire of being awake / I begin to wake. /

It gives me joy." Lisa Russ Spaar (ed.), *Acquainted With the Night: Insomnia Poems* (New York: Columbia University Press, 2019).

12:00
Unprocessed Emotions

1   The part that lights up when watching the video clip is called the emotional (or medial limbic) circuit. It comprises the areas of the brain related to emotions. "Good" sleepers can subsequently process these emotions. If you let them sleep for a night after watching the video and put them in the scanner again the next day, their brain reacts very differently when they see the same clip again; this time, there is much less reaction, and what reaction there is appears in different places. Interview with Eus van Someren (20 February 2019).

2   Part of this research can be found here: Rick Wassing et al., "Restless REM Sleep Impedes Overnight Amygdala Adaptation," *Current Biology*, Vol. 29, No. 14 (22 July 2019), pp. 2351–2358.

3   See also: Rick Wassing et al., "Slow Dissolving of Emotional Distress Contributes to Hyperarousal," *PNAS*, Vol. 113, No. 9 (1 March 2016), pp. 2538–2543.

4 An American doctor named Murray Raskind, who worked with a lot of war veterans, coincidentally discovered that a drug used to treat high blood pressure, which has the unintended side effect of suppressing noradrenaline, normalizes REM sleep in traumatized veterans with post-traumatic stress disorder (PTSD). When the veterans were relieved of their unstable REM sleep, they had far fewer nightmares and fewer other PTSD symptoms. See Walker, *Why We Sleep*, chapter 10.

13:00
Insomnia, Anxiety, and Depression

1 Having these genes is not a one-way ticket to insomnia. Genes do not irrevocably condemn you to nights spent tossing and turning; at most they give you a certain susceptibility to it. Whether or not this comes to light depends, for the main part, on the context: your experiences and your environment. It is virtually impossible to overestimate the influence of this.

2 Melancholy and disturbed sleep have traditionally gone hand in hand. For example, as early as 1621, the British doctor Robert Burton wrote in his extensive study *The Anatomy of Melancholy*, "Waking, by reason of their continual cares, fears, sorrows, is a symptom that much crucifies melancholy men."

3 People with depression wake up more often and have greater difficulty falling asleep. Their "sleep architecture" is also different; while NREM is usually deepest in the first sleep phase, it is deepest in the second phase for people with depression. They have very few deep sleep waves (phases 3 and 4 of the sleep cycle). However, it is mainly the REM sleep that appears to be disturbed. Some people with depression—this figure is as high as 40 percent among young people with depression—suffer from hypersomnia: the urge to sleep for a very long time. All in all, approximately 90 percent of people with depression also claim to have sleep problems. For an overview of decades of research into the relationship between sleep problems and depression, see: N. Tsuno et al., "Sleep and Depression," *Journal of Clinical Psychiatry*, Vol. 66, No. 10 (2005), pp. 1254–1269. See also: David Nutt et al., "Sleep Disorders as Core Symptoms of Depression," *Dialogues in Clinical Neuroscience*, Vol. 1, No. 3

(September 2008), pp. 329–336. For the complex connection between psychological complaints and sleep, see: Andrew Krystal, "Psychiatric Disorders and Sleep," *Neurologic Clinics*, Vol. 30, No. 4 (2012), pp. 1389–1413.

4 Vaughn McCall and Carmen Black, "The Link Between Suicide and Insomnia: Theoretical Mechanisms," *Current Psychiatry Reports*, Vol. 15, No. 9 (2013), p. 389.

5 The ideal scientific research looks at a single variable, meaning that all *other* factors must remain the same. For example, if you want to look at the influence that drinking coffee has on sleep, it is important that your test subjects don't suddenly change their diurnal rhythms, start taking their smartphones to bed, or start doing other things that could also influence their sleep. In those cases, you would not be able to deduce what influence the *coffee* had.

6 These include discovering various "diagnoses" or "subtypes" among insomniacs. These can't simply be summarized, à la "the depressive insomniac" or "the neurotic insomniac." The causes of sleep problems are too complex for this.

However, if you analyze old test results with these subtypes at your disposal, you find that some test groups, due to the strict inclusion criteria, consisted entirely of two or three subtypes, while the rest were excluded. It is therefore not such a surprise that the test results were often inconsistent. See also: "Slapeloosheid heeft vele gezichten," The Dutch Brain Institute (8 January 2019).

14:00
Sleep and Mood

1 "Insomniacs Unable to Get Emotional Distress Off Their Mind," The Dutch Brain Institute (26 April 2019).

2 Here, Meerlo is probably referring to Naomi Breslau et al., "Sleep Disturbance and Psychiatric Disorders: An Epidemiological Study of Young Adults," *Biological Psychiatry*, Vol. 39, No. 6 (15 March 1996), pp. 411–418. This study followed about a thousand people in their twenties in Michigan, and concluded that those who reported sleep problems in their first interview in 1989 were four times more likely to be depressed three years later. Other long-term studies also found that

sleep problems often develop prior to severe depression. See: "Sleep and Mental Health," *Harvard Mental Health Letter* (18 March 2019). Sleep problems are therefore diagnosed sooner, in any case, than the depression they announce. It is unclear whether they also *cause* the depression; perhaps they both stem from the same source. In that case, an unnamed problem X initially expresses itself as sleep problems and, if nothing is done about it, it grows into depression.

3   "The amygdala is usually inhibited by the regulatory part of your brain, the prefrontal cortex. This generally ensures that the emotions we feel, and which are generated by the amygdala, correspond to the situation in which we find ourselves. However, the prefrontal cortex is very sensitive to sleep deprivation. Even just one bad night is enough to make it less active. This means that the amygdala's 'brake' doesn't work very well, which causes you to overreact," Meerlo explains. This can also manifest itself in aggression. "Forensic psychologists, such as my colleague Marieke Lancel, note that psychiatric patients in secure units often

have sleep problems. These people also often say, 'I can feel whenever problems are imminent, because those are the periods in which I sleep badly.'"

4   A tried-and-true way of keeping rats awake is to put them on a small platform in a water tank, which regularly disappears under water. They have to keep moving in order not to drown, so they have to stay awake. Another method is to put them in a wheel that never stops turning. In both instances, the rats can't get any sleep. However, researchers accept that it is not possible to say whether the consequences of this treatment can be attributed to that lack of sleep, or also stress, the fear of death, and fatigue. See: Valeria Colavito et al., "Experimental Sleep Deprivation as a Tool to Test Memory Deficits in Rodents," *Frontiers in Systems Neuroscience*, Vol. 7, No. 106 (December 2013).

5   See: Peter Franzen and Daniel Buysse, "Sleep Disturbances and Depression: Risk Relationships for Subsequent Depression and Therapeutic Implications," *Dialogues in Clinical Neuroscience*, Vol. 10, No. 4 (2008), pp. 473–481.

6   Hong Fang et al., "Depression in Sleep Disturbance: A Review on a Bidirectional Relationship, Mechanisms and Treatment," *Journal of Cellular and Molecular Medicine*, Vol. 23, No. 4 (April 2019), pp. 2324–2332.

7   Unfortunately, it was not possible to have these things measured to see whether these aspects of my brain are abnormal.

8   In a press release from the Dutch Brain Institute about its research, which I already quoted above, they write: "Insomnia could primarily be caused by a failing neutralization of emotional distress. Which makes it understandable that insomnia is the primary risk factor for the development of disorders of mood, anxiety, and post-traumatic stress." See: "Insomniacs Unable to Get Emotional Distress Off Their Mind," The Dutch Brain Institute (26 April 2019).

9   You could ask yourself why this pain has to be as intense as it is in a depression, anxiety disorder, or insomnia. Could that signal not be a bit less vivid? In my experience, there is a point at which insomnia is self-perpetuating; that's usually when I am lying awake out

of fear of not sleeping. What started off as a useful response has then been derailed and ended up part of a vicious circle.

**15:00
Insomnia
Isn't Simply a Defect**

1   If you are less strict, and only ask who has trouble sleeping at least *once* per week, every week, the proportion of the population is as high as two in three, Walker (*Why We Sleep*, 2018) estimates. However, let's be strict. One in nine.

2   The figure in the Netherlands is one in ten. See: interview with Eus van Someren (20 February 2019). See also: "Slapeloosheid heeft vele gezichten," The Dutch Brain Institute (8 January 2019). Kerkhof's (2017) epidemiological study reports a rate of 9.5 percent clinical insomnia among Dutch women and 6.8 percent among men.

3   This is exactly what Walker claims. Real insomnia is a result of innate, biological factors that don't have anything to do with a person's environment: the "error" lies in the person themself. "External factors that cause poor sleep, such as too much

bright light at night, the wrong ambient room temperature, caffeine, tobacco, and alcohol consumption... can masquerade as insomnia. However, their origins are not from *within* you, and therefore not a disorder *of* you. Rather, they are influences from outside... Other factors, however, come from within a person, and are innate biological causes of insomnia."

4 According to Walker, insomnia is almost twice as prevalent in women as it is in men. See Walker, *Why We Sleep*, chapter 12. I have been unable to verify these figures; all of the studies I consulted reported that women suffer from insomnia more often than men, but the difference is usually less great; for example, more than a quarter of women compared to less than a fifth of men in America. See: Ronald Kessler et al., "Insomnia and the Performance of U.S. Workers: Results From the America Insomnia Survey," *Sleep*, Vol. 34, No. 9 (2011), pp. 1161–1171. Interestingly, data from the U.S. Centers for Disease Control and Prevention show women on average sleep slightly longer per night than men, despite their more common sleeping problems. CDC, "Short Sleep Duration Among U.S. Adults," accessed July 2022.

5 Almost 25 percent of Dutch people with an immigrant background report waking up not feeling rested, compared to 14 percent of white Dutch people. And while one in ten white Dutch people feel tired during the day, that applies to as many as one in four Dutch people with an immigrant background. This is from a large-scale meta-analysis of sleeping data from 135,519 Dutch people gleaned from thirty-four Dutch population surveys over the past twenty-five years, carried out by the Trimbos Institute. See: S. Leone et al., "Slechte slaap: een probleem voor de volksgezondheid?," Trimbos Institute (March 2018).

6 See: "What's the Connection Between Race and Sleep Disorders?," Sleep Foundation (30 July 2020). At least a third of the Latin American and African Americans surveyed indicated that they lay awake at least two nights per week due to financial worries, and worries about their work, health, or relationships. Among white Americans or Americans with Asian roots, this figure was almost

a quarter. This is based on research carried out by the American Sleep Foundation. See: "Poll Reveals Sleep Differences Among Ethnic Groups," Sleep Foundation (8 March 2010). The following study provides an overview of research that has so far been carried out into these differences: Dayna Johnson, "Are Sleep Patterns Influenced by Race/Ethnicity—a Marker of Relative Advantage or Disadvantage? Evidence to Date," *Nature and Science of Sleep*, Vol. 11 (2019), pp. 79–95.

7   For example, 33 percent of white Americans get fewer than the recommended seven hours of sleep per night, against 46 percent of Black or Native Hawaiian Americans, according to statistics from the Centers for Disease Control and Prevention, "Short Sleep Duration Among U.S. Adults," last updated in 2017; accessed July 2022.

8   Cees van den Boom, "Bijna een kwart van de Nederlanders heeft slaapproblemen," *Trouw* (20 August 2019).

9   No large-scale population studies into sleep among Dutch people have yet been carried out. See: Tomas van Dijk, "Steeds meer Nederlanders

kampen met slaapproblemen— klopt dit wel?," *de Volkskrant* (26 August 2019).

10   See: Maria Calem et al., "Increased Prevalence of Insomnia and Changes in Hypnotics Use in England Over 15 years: Analysis of the 1993, 2000, and 2007 National Psychiatric Morbidity Surveys," *Sleep*, Vol. 35, No. 3 (March 2012), pp. 377–384.

11   To be precise, from 11.9 to 15.5 percent. See: Ståle Pallesen et al., "A 10-Year Trend of Insomnia Prevalence in the Adult Norwegian Population," *Sleep Medicine*, Vol. 15, No. 2 (February 2014), pp. 173–179.

12   According to China Sleep Research Report 2022 as relayed by Lisa Nan, "China's One Trillion Yen Sleeping Economy," *Jing Daily* (7 April 2022).

13   Those aged eighteen to twenty-four reported a 31 percent growth in sleeping problems, those aged twenty-five to thirty-four a whopping 49 percent increase. E.S. Ford et al., "Trends in Insomnia and Excessive Daytime Sleepiness Among U.S. Adults From 2002 to 2012," *Sleep Medicine*, Vol. 16, No. 3 (March 2015), pp. 372–378.

14   Connor M. Sheehan et al., "Are U.S. Adults Reporting

Less Sleep? Findings From Sleep Duration Trends in the National Health Interview Survey, 2004–2017," *Sleep*, Vol. 42, No. 2 (February 2019).

15 It is very hard to assess long-term changes in sleep, because it was not regularly included in early cohort studies and health surveys until the 1980s; only recently has sleep started to attract much scholarly attention. Moreover, differences in measurement methods between studies make it hard to compare them and get firm numbers. Also, many studies depend on self-reported use of time, but have no way of checking whether time spent in bed is also spent asleep, and not texting or watching TV. For doubts about the reduction of American sleep time, see: R.P. Ogilvie and S.R. Patel, "Changing National Trends in Sleep Duration: Did We Make America Sleep Again?," *Sleep*, Vol. 41, No. 4 (April 2018). Some studies suggest *no* decline in sleep time. S.D. Youngstedt et al., "Has Adult Sleep Duration Declined Over the Last 50+ Years?," *Sleep Medicine Review*, Vol. 28, (August 2016), pp. 69–85.

16 For a helpful overview of different and sometimes conflicting research findings, see

Justin Fox, "Americans Are Sleeping More, If Not Necessarily Better," *Bloomberg* (28 July 2021).

17 Michael A. Grandner et al., "Declining Annual Trends in U.S. Daily Sleep Duration Are Greater Among Racial/Ethnic Minorities: Implications for Cardiometabolic Disease Disparities," *Circulation* (April 2022).

18 Market research bureau Statista reports this sharp rise in Nils-Gerrit Wunsch, "Sales of Melatonin in the U.S. 2008–2020," 29 November 2021. According to the Sleep Foundation, sales of melatonin supplements in the U.S. grew from $62 million in 2003 to $378 million in 2014, an increase of 500 percent. In 2020, 14.5 percent of U.S. adults had trouble falling asleep most days or every day in the past thirty days. See: NCHS Data Brief, No. 436 (June 2022).

19 According to the 2019 Philips Global Sleep Survey.

20 Hospital admissions for under sixteens with a primary diagnosis of sleep disorder rose from 6,549 in 2012–13 to 9,451 in 2017–18 to 11,313 in 2018–19. See: Sarah Marsh, "Sharp Rise in Hospital Admissions for Children With Sleep Disorders," *The Guardian* (6 March 2022).

21 Figures for the years 2002–2014 among Nordic youths show an increase in sleeping problems. See: E.B. Thorsteinsson et al., "Trends in Sleeping Difficulty Among Adolescents in Five Nordic Countries 2002–2014," *Nordic Welfare Research* (11 November 2019), pp. 77–87.

22 Some clinics report an increase by as much as 80 percent in referrals of secondary school pupils, and up to 50 percent in primary children. The exact time frame in which this increase has taken place is not clear from the reports. "80 procent meer middelbare scholieren verwezen naar slaappoli," *Een Vandaag* (30 November 2017).

23 Research carried out by Amsterdam's OLVG Hospital reveals that as many as 40 percent of Amsterdam residents between the ages of twenty and forty have sleep problems. That is twice as high as the figures from Statistics Netherlands suggest for the same age cohort. See: "Onderzoek OLVG: Amsterdamse millennial slaapt slecht," OLVG (10 October 2019).

24 "The burden of depression and other mental health conditions is on the rise globally," the WHO writes in its "Fact Sheet on Depression" (30 January 2020).

Over fifty years, the number of suicides has increased by 60 percent. Between 1988 and 2008, the use of antidepressants in America increased by 400 percent. See: T.M. Luhrmann, "Is the World More Depressed?," *New York Times* (24 March 2014). That is consistent with figures from the United Kingdom, for example, which show a huge increase in anxiety disorders. Since 2008, the percentage of young adults with severe anxiety symptoms has tripled. This is particularly prevalent among young women. Anxiety symptoms among other age groups have also increased significantly. See: Denis Campbell, "U.K. Has Experienced 'Explosion' in Anxiety Since 2008, Study Finds," *The Guardian* (14 September 2020). See also: April Slee et al., "Trends in Generalised Anxiety Disorders and Symptoms in Primary Care: U.K. Population-Based Cohort Study," *British Journal of Psychiatry*, Vol. 218, No. 3 (2020), pp. 158–164.

25 After all, the brain is extremely plastic, and changes depending on the way in which it is used and nurtured. See: Margreet Fogteloo and Casper Thomas, "Gymnastiek voor het plastische brein," *De Groene Amsterdammer* (16 November 2011).

26 K.M. Zitting et al., "Google Trends Reveals Increases in Internet Searches for Insomnia During the 2019 Coronavirus Disease (COVID-19) Global Pandemic," *Journal of Sleep Medicine* (1 February 2021).

27 See: Express Scripts, "America's State of Mind Report: Use of Mental Health Medications Increasing With Spread of Coronavirus" (16 April 2020).

28 R. Robillard et al., "Profiles of Sleep Changes During the COVID-19 Pandemic: Demographic, Behavioural and Psychological Factors," *Journal of Sleep Research*, Vol. 30, No. 1 (2021).

29 For instance, some evidence is emerging of mental health problems like PTSD and severe insomnia in post-COVID patients. See: S. El Sayed et al., "Sleep in Post-COVID-19 Recovery Period and Its Impact on Different Domains of Quality of Life," *Egyptian Journal of Neurology, Psychiatry and Neurosurgery*, Vol. 57, No. 1 (2021), p. 172.

30 Economic uncertainty, such as that caused by the coronavirus crisis, is one of the factors known to be detrimental to sleep. Read more about this in chapter 20:00.

31 Even neuroscientists acknowledge the key role of emotions in the development of insomnia, though they refer to it as "cognitive-emotional hyperarousal." If you are emotionally hyperactive, or experience strong emotions, you are more likely to lie awake as a result, researchers conclude. See: Julio Fernández-Mendoza et al., "Cognitive-Emotional Hyperarousal as a Premorbid Characteristic of Individuals Vulnerable to Insomnia," *Psychosomatic Medicine*, Vol. 72, No. 4 (May 2010), pp. 397–403.

32 Walker writes in *Why We Sleep*: "The two most common triggers of chronic insomnia are psychological: (1) emotional concerns, or worry, and (2) emotional distress, or anxiety."

33 Walker, *Why We Sleep*.

34 The idea that a "disorder" is perhaps not a meaningless defect, but a meaningful response to a defective situation, is convincingly substantiated in *Lost Connections*, the book that journalist Johann Hari wrote following his own long-standing experiences with depression. When he discovers that depression is actually *not* a case of too little serotonin, like he always thought, he starts

researching the societal developments and living conditions that contribute to the development of depression. He uses an array of studies to show that a lack of meaningful work, a lack of meaningful values, a lack of human contact, a lack of nature, a lack of future prospects, and a lack of economic certainty all contribute to the development of depression. Or anxiety, as all of these factors also contribute to anxiety disorders. Do they also contribute to the development of insomnia? Hari doesn't mention that, and when I investigated it, it appeared that in most cases too little research has been carried out to make an authoritative statement (the exceptions can be found in the notes at the end of this book). However, Hari's study is also very interesting for insomniacs: since depression almost always goes hand in hand with sleeping problems, it seems perfectly possible that many of the proven causes that Hari identifies for depression are also relevant to insomnia. See: Johann Hari, *Lost Connections: Why You're Depressed and How to Find Hope* (London: Bloomsbury, 2018).

16:00 Sleep in the Spotlight

1   See the book *Identiteit* by Paul Verhaeghe (Amsterdam: De Bezige Bij, 2012) for more information about this. Verhaeghe looks in detail at the conviction that everything needs a scientific explanation. He refers to this as "scientism."

2   There is certainly a way to include the (social) context, namely by carrying out epidemiological research. This is when a phenomenon such as insomnia is not investigated on an individual level, but on the level of the entire population: How prevalent is it? Is it linked to other factors such as age, gender, income, etc.? However, epidemiological research doesn't offer any scope for the specific, complex situation of all those individuals insofar as it doesn't fall into those big denominators.

3   Verhaeghe, *Identiteit.*

4   For more information about first and second sleep, see the study by Roger Ekirch, which unearthed this forgotten phenomenon: *At Day's Close: A History of Nighttime* (London: W&N, 2006).

5   See, for example: Bastiaan Nagtegaal, "RIVM: kinderen

slapen slecht door het licht van hun telefoons," NRC *Handelsblad* (6 March 2019).

6 Some studies have shown that bright light keeps you up longer at night, but participants in such studies were wearing diving masks with LEDs in them, for example—not a particularly good representation of the light from your phone, *de Volkskrant* writes in a fact-check about blue light. See: Maarten Keulemans, "Nee, het blauwe licht van uw schermpjes is níet wat u wakker houdt," *de Volkskrant* (10 May 2019).

7 Researchers concluded this from a systematic review of ninety studies on this topic. See: Lauren Hale et al., "Screen Time and Sleep Among School-Aged Children and Adolescents: A Systematic Literature Review," *Sleep Medicine Reviews*, Vol. 21 (June 2015), pp. 50–58. A survey of four thousand Brits carried out by consultancy firm Deloitte revealed that half of young people check their phones in the middle of the night. Throughout the entire population, this figure was one in three. This was in 2016. The use of phones has only increased since then. See: "There's No Place Like Phone," Deloitte (2016).

8 After all, the brain is extremely plastic, and changes depending on the way in which it is used. Babies, for example, develop a brain that best fits their environment. See: Mark Miears, "De ontwikkelingen in het babybrein," *Psychologie Magazine* (17 March 2020).

17:00 You Feel More Than You Feel You Do

1 Originally published in Dutch as "Zoals," *Zoals* (Amsterdam: Uitgeverij de Harmonie, 1992). Translation taken from: Judith Herzberg, *But What: Selected Poems*, translated by Shirley Kaufman with Judith Herzberg, Field Translation Series 13 (1988), p. 109.

2 This is what Robert Stickgold, sleep researcher at Harvard thinks, for example. See, also for the previous two paragraphs: Alice Robb, *Why We Dream: The Transformative Power of Our Nightly Journey* (London: Pan Macmillan, 2018).

3 If you *were* to become aware of these affects—and recognize and name them as specific emotions—that could make a difference. Emotions, and the underlying affects, are related to tension, Verhaeghe explains. "If you become aware of these

affects, you may be able to control this tension in a certain way. It could even be the case that simply the fact that you are aware of a certain tension changes the course of that tension. We know too little about this to draw firm conclusions."

4   If you would rather stay clear of anything that has too strong a whiff of incense, walking (without the distraction of headphones or smartphone) is also a good way to "land" in your body. See: Bregje Hofstede, *De herontdekking van het lichaam* (Amsterdam: Cossee, 2016).

5   The series, by Fokke Obbema, was collected and published as: *De zin van het leven: gesprekken over de essentie van ons bestaan* (Amsterdam: Atlas Contact, 2019). For my interview, see: Fokke Obbema, "Schrijfster Bregje Hofstede: 'Het leven is een dunne draad over een complete leegte,'" *de Volkskrant* (16 December 2018).

18:00
Dreams as a Way to Access Emotions

1   The Bible reads, "[God] speaks in dreams, in visions of the night, when deep sleep falls on people as they lie in their beds. He whispers in their ears." The Quran also attaches meaning to dreams, and the Muslim call to prayer, the adhan, was apparently inspired by a dream that one of Mohammed's contemporaries had. For Tibetan Buddhists, being awake is actually the lowest form of awareness; sleeping and dreaming are higher up the spiritual ladder. See: Robb, *Why We Dream*.

2   The strength of the Greek belief in the connection between dreams and illness can also be seen in the figure of the god Asclepius, who was the god of dreams *and* healing. If you were unwell, you could invoke him, and if you were lucky you would receive instructions for your treatment in your dreams. See: Robb, *Why We Dream*.

3   Ibid.

4   See: Walker, *Why We Sleep*.

5   See: R. Cartwright, "Dreams That Work: The Relation of Dream Incorporation to Adaptation to Stressful Events," *Dreaming*, Vol. 1, No. 1 (1991), pp. 3–9. And: Matteo Maillard, "Rêver de son échec à un examen aiderait à sa réussite," *Le Monde* (14 November 2014). Both studies are referred to in Robb, *Why We Dream*.

6   "It may also mean that you struggle holding onto things,"

according to the "dream symbol library" at GroteBeer.net.

7   Robb, *Why We Dream*.

8   Oliver Sacks, *Awakenings* (New York: Vintage, 2013 [1973]).

9   Robb, *Why We Dream*.

10 Figures from the Netherlands do indicate a recent decline in use. The government is also pursuing a policy to discourage their use. See: "Sterke afname gebruik benzodiazepinen," *Pharmaceutisch Weekblad*, Vol. 115, No. 44 (29 October 2020).

11 These figures are taken from Walker, *Why We Sleep*.

12 A quote from the American author Henry James, which may be apocryphal since it is also sometimes attributed to Lawrence Sanders.

19:00
Context

1   "A person's mental health and many common mental disorders are shaped by various social, economic, and physical environments operating at different stages of life." See: WHO and the Calouste Gulbenkian Foundation, *Social Determinants of Mental Health* (2014). Quoted in: Hari, *Lost Connections*.

2   On World Health Day 2017, the UN stated that "the dominant biomedical narrative of depression [is based on] biased and selective use of research outcomes [that] must be abandoned." Instead, "social problems" and "power imbalances" deserve greater attention. Quoted in: Johann Hari, "Is Everything You Think You Know About Depression Wrong?," *The Guardian* (7 January 2018).

3   It is well known that social inequality is very stressful and contributes to stress-related disorders. Paul Verhaeghe clearly outlines the extensive scientific research related to the connection between society and mental health in his book *Identiteit*. With regard to depression, I would recommend Johann Hari's book *Lost Connections*.

4   Higher temperatures make it much more difficult to sleep well. It is therefore expected that climate change, apart from being disastrous for the world, will also be bad for our sleep in the short term and that older and poorer people will be worst affected. See: Nick Obradovich et al., "Nighttime Temperature and Human Sleep Loss in a Changing Climate," *Science Advances*, Vol. 3, No. 5 (2017).

20:00
Money

1   See: Emma Bedford, "Global Market Value of the Sleep Economy From 2019 to 2024," Statista (25 May 2020). This relates to products, services, and apps designed to help consumers sleep.

2   See: ReportLinker, *Global Book Publishing Industry Market Report* (July 2020). Market research company IbisWorld also estimates it is worth around $110 billion per year. ResearchAndMarkets estimates a more modest $92 billion.

3   McKinsey estimates turnover of $40 billion in the U.S. alone, and growth of more than 8 percent per year. See: Dan Goldman, "Investing in the Growing Sleep-Health Economy," McKinsey & Company (30 August 2017).

4   The privacy education website Common Sense Privacy Program writes that the predecessor, Pokémon Go, collected and was able to sell all sorts of personal information, including geolocation, first name and surname, email address and telephone number, and postal address. Add sleep information to the mix and you can easily target the users with all sorts of products aimed at improving sleep, for example.

Pokémon Go generated $2 billion in profits for the inventors, in part through advertising income, and in part because the monsters didn't just appear anywhere at random: companies could buy "hotspots," meaning that players ended up at places like McDonald's or Starbucks while looking for Pokémon. See: Gareth Damian Martin, "How Pokémon Sleep Promises to Commodify Our Dreams," *Frieze* (13 June 2019).

5   Kaitlyn Wylde, "What Does Having a Boyfriend Have to Do With Sleep?," *New York Times* (2 October 2019).

6   Walker lists a number of these gadgets. There is a gadget, for example, that is designed to improve your memory by 40 percent the next morning by playing tick-tock sounds synchronized with your personal brainwaves. There are also electrodes that pulse in time with your deep sleep waves, claimed to double the number of facts you are able to recall. Supersonic sleep for extra intelligence is already attainable to those with a lot of money. Walker warns of products you can order online that may cause burns. Walker, *Why We Sleep*, chapter 6.

7   From the website meetsomnox.nl.

8   From the website zekerslapen.nl.

9   Ibid.

10 Ibid.

11 Of the 20 percent of Dutch people with the lowest income, 28 percent have sleep problems. Of the 20 percent with the highest income, that percentage is almost half as much. See: Statistics Netherlands, "Een op de vijf meldt slaapproblemen" (16 March 2018).

12 M.A. Grandner et al., "Who Gets the Best Sleep? Ethnic and Socioeconomic Factors Related to Sleep Complaints," *Sleep Medicine*, Vol. 11, No. 5 (May 2010), pp. 470–478. See also: M.A. Grandner et al., "Sleep Disparity, Race/Ethnicity, and Socioeconomic Position," *Sleep Medicine*, Vol. 18 (February 2016), pp. 7–18.

13 In the U.S., the median family income for those with no high school diploma is $22,320, while those with an advanced degree generally earn $116,265—which is more than five times as much. See: Scott A. Wolla and Jessica Sullivan, "Education, Income and Wealth," Economic Research, Federal Reserve Bank of St. Louis (January 2017).

14 Of Dutch people with the highest level of education, 21.8 percent have sleep problems, whereas those with the lowest level of education have the highest percentage of sleep problems: 38.4 percent. See Kerkhof, "Epidemiology of Sleep and Sleep Disorders in the Netherlands."

15 Francesco Cappuccio et al., "The Sociology of Sleep," *Sleep, Health, and Society: From Aetiology to Public Health* (Oxford: Oxford University Press, 2018). In a different study of 160,000 Americans, those without a high school diploma were 1.8 times more likely to have sleep problems than the average college graduate. See: Michael Grandner et al., "Who Gets the Best Sleep? Ethnic and Socioeconomic Factors Related to Sleep Complaints," *Sleep Medicine*, Vol. 11, No. 5 (May 2010), pp. 470–478.

16 See: M.A. Grandner et al., "Who Gets the Best Sleep?"

17 See: Nirav P. Patel et al., "'Sleep Disparity' in the Population: Poor Sleep Quality Is Strongly Associated With Poverty and Ethnicity," BMC *Public Health*, Vol. 10 (2010), p. 475.

18 Kriston McIntosh et al., "Examining the Black-White Wealth Gap," Brookings (27 February 2020). "Right now the net wealth of a typical Black family in America is around one-tenth that of a white family," writes Liz Mineo in "Racial Wealth Gap May Be a Key to Other Inequalities," *Harvard Gazette* (3 June 2021).

19 See: Aditya Aladangady and Akila Forde, "Wealth Inequality and the Racial Wealth Gap," FEDS notes (21 October 2021).

20 For a meta-analysis of recent research into this topic, see M.A. Grandner et al., "Sleep Disparity, Race/Ethnicity, and Socioeconomic Position," *Sleep Medicine*, Vol. 18 (February 2016), pp. 7–18.

21 See: M.A. Grandner, "Sleep, Health, and Society," *Sleep Medicine Clinics*, Vol. 12, No. 1 (2017), pp. 1–22. "A rigorous 2015 study involving both lab tests and self-reports from more than 2,000 U.S. participants found that, compared with whites matched for age and sex, Blacks were five times as likely to sleep for shorter periods. Hispanics and Chinese Americans were roughly two times as likely to get fewer hours of sleep than whites."

See: Katherine Ellison, The Great Sleep Divide," *Knowable Magazine* (7 March 2021).

22 PRB, "A Demographic Profile of U.S. Workers Around the Clock" (18 September 2008).

23 I write "women," and not "womxn" or a different term that allows for non-binary or transgender people because the research I refer to does not make that distinction: it only relates to cis women. Sleep problems prominently affect transgender and non-binary people and are (to a limited extent) researched separately. See, for example: Salem Harry-Hernandez et al., "Gender Dysphoria, Mental Health, and Poor Sleep Health Among Transgender and Gender Non-binary Individuals: A Qualitative Study in New York City," *Transgender Health*, Vol. 5, No. 1 (16 March 2020), pp. 59–68.

24 According to figures from Statistics Netherlands from 2018. Some researchers, including Walker, report *twice as many* insomnia diagnoses for women.

25 A large meta-study reviewing multiple large epidemiological studies from North America, Europe, Asia, and Africa found women run about 58 percent

more risk of insomnia. L.N. Zeng et al., "Gender Difference in the Prevalence of Insomnia: A Meta-Analysis of Observational Studies," *Frontiers in Psychiatry* (20 November 2020). An earlier meta-study from 2006 found a 41 percent higher risk for women. See: Bin Zhang and Yun-Kwok Wing, "Sex Differences in Insomnia: A Meta-Analysis," *Sleep*, Vol. 29, No. 1 (2006), pp. 85–93.

26 Kessler et al., "Insomnia and the Performance of U.S. Workers."

27 The gender difference reported in the Netherlands is greatest during puberty. See: Kerkhof, "Epidemiology of Sleep and Sleep Disorders in the Netherlands."

28 The difference is smaller among men and women who report sleeping badly "some of the time." See: Ashleigh J. Rich et al., "Gender/Sex Disparity in Self-Reported Sleep Quality Among Canadian Adults," *UBC Medical Journal*, Vol. 11, No. 2 (2020), pp. 11–16. According to Statistics Canada health reports from 2017, Canadian women report sleeping somewhat longer but have more difficulty falling or staying asleep than men, with 43 percent of

men and 55 percent of women reporting sleeping problems.

29 This was the conclusion based on research among more than eight thousand Brits. See: Sara Arber, "Gender, Marital Status and Sleep Problems in Britain," *Przegl Lek*, Vol. 69, No. 2 (2012), pp. 54–60. Others seek the explanation for the difference in the "double societal burden" of women who still shoulder more unpaid labor next to their paid jobs. See: Peter Vantyghem, "Vrouwen slapen niet zolekker als mannen," *De Standaard* (25 September 2015).

30 Compared to two in ten men. See: Daniël Herbers and Wil Portegijs, "Hoeveel vrouwen zijn economisch zelfstandig?," *Emancipatiemonitor CBS/SCP* (14 December 2018).

31 See: Lien van der Leij, "Waar is mijn drie ton gebleven?," *Het Financieele Dagblad* (29 March 2014). These figures are based on research by WomenInc.

32 European Union, Factsheet on the Gender Pay Gap, "Equal Pay? Time to Close the Gap" (October 2021).

33 Amanda Barroso and Anna Brown, "Gender Pay Gap in U.S. Held Steady in 2020," Pew Research Center (25 May 2021).

34　This applies to Black women who work full-time, year-round, as compared to their non-Hispanic white male counterparts; a great pay gap persists across educational levels and occupations. See these calculations by the National Women's Law Center: Brandie Temple and Jasmine Tucker, "Equal Pay for Black Women" (27 July 2017).

35　Pamela Duncan, "U.K. Gender Pay Gap: Women Paid 90p for £1 Earned by Men," *The Guardian* (6 April 2022).

36　See: Dustin T. Duncan, Ichiro Kawachi, and Susan Redline (eds.), *The Social Epidemiology of Sleep* (Oxford: Oxford University Press, 2019), chapter 10. In fact, there is some evidence that higher household income is also associated with more insufficient sleep, suggesting some high earners are trading sleep for extra income; but this effect only becomes apparent when you adjust for covariates like education, occupation, healthcare, mental health, age, gender, ethnicity, household size, employment status, healthy diet, body mass index, and other factors which are often connected to income.

37　Income and health are closely connected. See, for example,

these figures from the National Institute for Public Health and the Environment (RIVM): "Sociaaleconomische status en gezondheid," Volksgezondheidenzorg.info (2020).

38　The poet Dana Gioia articulates it wonderfully in "Insomnia." "Now you hear what the house has to say. / Pipes clanking, water running in the dark, / the mortgaged walls shifting in discomfort / [...] the murmur of property, of things in disrepair, / the moving parts about to come undone."

39　That is shown by research from the University of Pennsylvania. See: Michael Grandner et al., "Sleep Symptoms, Race/Ethnicity, and Socioeconomic Position," *Journal of Clinical Sleep Medicine*, Vol. 9, No. 9 (15 September 2013), pp. 897–905.

40　There is even a sleep disorder called "shift work disorder," which is a condition that affects people who work such varying shifts. See: Danielle Pacheco and Abhinav Singh, "Shift Work Disorder Symptoms," Sleep Foundation (16 October 2020). Night shifts are also very bad for your sleep quality. People who work night shifts are more than twice as likely to suffer from severe sleep disturbance. See: Valéria de Castilho Palhares et al., "Association Between Sleep Quality and Quality of Life in Nursing Professionals Working Rotating Shifts," *Revista de Saude Publica*, Vol. 48, No. 4 (2014), pp. 594–601.

41 Of Dutch people who have attended a vocational college or university, 3.8 percent regularly work night shifts, as opposed to 10.2 percent of those who have general secondary education or secondary vocational education as their highest level of education. That is according to the Monitor Arbeid 2017 from TNO. See: "NEQ Benchmarktool werktijden," *Nationale Enquête Arbeidsomstandigheden TNO/CBS* (2019). In the Netherlands, 53.6 percent of people sometimes work in the evening; more than a quarter do so regularly. Approximately 10 percent of Dutch people regularly work at night. And more than two thirds do overtime, according to the *Nationale Enquête Arbeidsomstandigheden* (2018). The international figures are similar: less than a quarter of European employees have a regular, nine-to-five job. See: G. Costa et al., "Flexible Working Hours, Health, and Well-Being in Europe: Some Considerations From a SALTSA Project," *Chronobiology International*, Vol. 21 (2004), pp. 831–844. A fifth of European employees sometimes work night shifts, with 10 percent doing so more than five times a month. See: "5th European Working Condition Survey."

42 This is the conclusion of the International Agency for Research on Cancer, part of the World Health Organization. See: "Night Shift Work," *IARC Monographs on the Identification of Carcinogenic Hazards to Humans*, Vol. 124 (2019).

43 Among Dutch people. See: Kerkhof, "Epidemiology of Sleep and Sleep Disorders in the Netherlands." A large international study found that sleep issues move in parallel with the unemployment rate, both increasing at the same time, and that the long-term unemployed especially suffer from disturbed sleep. See: David Blanchflower and Alex Bryson, "Unemployment and Sleep: Evidence From the United States and Europe," *Economics & Human Biology*, Vol. 43 (13 July 2021), 101042.

44 Read more about universal basic income in Hari's *Lost Connections* or Rutger

Bregman, *Gratis geld voor iedereen* (Amsterdam: De Correspondent, 2014).

45 The researchers report a "major improvement in quality of sleep." See: "Report on the Preliminary Results of the B-Mincome Project (2017–2018): Combining a Guaranteed Minimum Income and Active Social Policies in Deprived Urban Areas of Barcelona," *Ajuntament de Barcelona* (July 2019), p. 38. For Mincome, see: Evelyn Forget, "The Basic Income Path to a Healthier Society," *Glasgow Centre for Population Health* (5 October 2018).

46 On average, the living costs of tenants in the Netherlands amount to 38.1 percent of their income, and for homeowners, that figure is 29 percent. Compared to 2012, the living costs have increased by about 12 percent, but they have remained stable for the last couple of years. This is shown in figures from Statistics Netherlands. "Woonlasten ten opzichte inkomen niet verder gestegen," Statistics Netherlands (4 April 2019). In Belgium too, living costs form the greatest expense for households. More than 30 percent of the household budget goes on living

costs. Twenty years ago, that was approximately 26 percent. See: "Huisvesting neemt steeds grotere hap uit huishoudbudget," *Statbel* (28 December 2019).

47 See: Vicky Robin, *Your Money or Your Life: 9 Steps to Transforming Your Relationship With Money and Achieving Financial Independence* (New York: Penguin, 2007).

48 It is not by chance that this is the title of the FIRE bible mentioned in the note above.

49 This realization is not only based on the FIRE movement, but also on the concept of "time banks." These are platforms where you can barter on the basis of time, instead of money. The currency is hours. You can exchange one "time bank hour" of your bookkeeping skills for an hour of a handyman, for example. Time is actually a more honest currency than money, as a day has twenty-four hours regardless of how rich or poor you are. This concept is not new—"time notes" were already circulating in the United Kingdom at the beginning of the nineteenth century, to the value of one or several hours' work—but it is currently making a comeback. Brussels and The Hague already have

"time banks," online platforms where you can do business with your time, and one is to be launched in Amsterdam soon.

21:00
Time

1   I wrote earlier that sleep complaints increased significantly during the pandemic, but that didn't apply to everyone. Those who had a secure income perhaps enjoyed being able to have a lie-in all of a sudden. The headline from the NRC on 28 April 2020 focused on this disparity: "Nachtrust in de coronacrisis: de één slaapt beter dan ooit, de ander doet geen oog dicht." (Sleep in the coronavirus crisis: some people are sleeping better than ever, while others aren't getting a wink.)

2   In total, eight in ten of those surveyed were unsatisfied with their sleep, and four in ten had sleep problems. See: "Onderzoek OLVG: Amsterdamse millennial slaapt slecht," OLVG (10 October 2019).

3   Torbjörn Åkerstedt et al., "Work Load and Work Hours in Relation to Disturbed Sleep and Fatigue in a Large Representative Sample," *Journal of Psychosomatic Research*, Vol. 53, No. 1 (2002), pp. 585–588. See

also: Torbjörn Åkerstedt, "Psychosocial Stress and Impaired Sleep," *Scandinavian Journal of Work, Environment & Health*, Vol. 32, No. 6 (2007), pp. 493–501.

4   See: H. Knudsen et al., "Job Stress and Poor Sleep Quality: Data From an American Sample of Full-Time Workers," *Social Science & Medicine*, Vol. 64, No. 10 (2007).

5   See: Åkerstedt, "Psychosocial Stress and Impaired Sleep."

6   A longitudinal study of 20,000 French employees showed that those who always had to rush, had to do several things at once, or were often interrupted were significantly more likely to suffer from psychological complaints and sleep problems. Working weeks of more than forty-eight hours and shift work certainly didn't help, but it was time pressure that emerged as one of the major risk factors for the development of sleep problems. See: C. Ribet and F. Derriennic, "Age, Working Conditions, and Sleep Disorders: A Longitudinal Analysis in the French Cohort E.S.T.E.V.," *Sleep: Journal of Sleep Research & Sleep Medicine*, Vol. 22, No. 4 (1999), pp. 491–504.

7   A study of 760 Australian nurses also revealed that a

high work pace leads to serious stress and fatigue. Those who had to work at high speed found their work not so much physically as psychologically taxing, and that psychological pressure led to worse sleep. A hectic work pace was therefore much more likely to go hand in hand with serious stress and exhaustion. It was not so much the duration as the quality of the nurses' sleep that suffered, which means that they recovered less well per hour slept, which led to the exhaustion. See: Peter Winwood and Kurt Lushington, "Disentangling the Effects of Psychological and Physical Work Demands on Sleep, Recovery and Maladaptive Chronic Stress Outcomes Within a Large Sample of Australian Nurses," *Journal of Advanced Nursing*, Vol. 56, No. 6 (December 2006), pp. 679–689.

8   Time pressure is a major predictive factor for disturbed sleep, and in the long term for sick leave and burnout. See: Christine Syrek and Conny Antoni, "Unfinished Tasks Foster Rumination and Impair Sleeping, Especially If Leaders Have High Performance Expectations," *Journal of Occupational Health Psychology*, Vol. 19, No. 4 (October 2014), pp. 490–499.

9   Ibid. See also: Martial Berset et al., "Work Stressors and Impaired Sleep: Rumination as a Mediator," *Stress and Health*, Vol. 27, No. 2 (April 2011), pp. 71–82.

10   I referred to the research about this in an article for *De Correspondent*. See: Bregje Hofstede, "Hoe je je wél aan je goede voornemens kunt houden," *De Correspondent* (1 January 2017).

11   If you wish to change your working week in the hope of getting more sleep, it may be interesting to know that the amount of work you have to complete is not the only issue. The type of work can also promote or detract from the quality of your sleep. Work that is repetitive and that you don't have much autonomy over often goes hand in hand with poor sleep (and also with depression). Work that is never really finished is also stressful and can keep you up at night. See Syrek and Antoni, "Unfinished Tasks Foster Rumination and Impair Sleeping."

12   See: Hofstede, "Hoe je je wél aan je goede voornemens kunt houden."

22:00
Place

1 The technology in your smartphone is *designed* to remove you from time and place. Thanks to the smartphone you can speak to people, work, or manage your finances at any place and time. See: Bregje Hofstede, "Hoe de smartphone van de hele wereld een wachtkamer maakt," *De Correspondent* (14 September 2016).

2 See for example: "Tel Aviv Trials 'Zombie' Traffic Lights to Save Smartphone Users From Themselves," *Times of Israel* (6 March 2019).

3 George Sturt, *Change in the Village* (Cambridge: Cambridge University Press, 2010).

4 The villagers used to only go there for special things such as sea salt or iron ore, which they couldn't make, cultivate, or find in their surrounding environment.

5 Sturt, *Change in the Village*.

6 Michael Norton et al., "The 'IKEA Effect': When Labor Leads to Love," *Journal of Consumer Psychology*, Vol. 22, No. 3 (July 2012), pp. 453–460.

7 Robert Zajonc, "Attitudinal Effects of Mere Exposure," *Journal of Personality and Social Psychology*, Vol. 9, No. 2 (1968), pp. 1–27.

8 Daniel Kahneman et al., "Anomalies: The Endowment Effect, Loss Aversion, and Status Quo Bias," *Journal of Economic Perspectives*, Vol. 5, No. 1 (1991), pp. 193–206.

9 Quing Li et al., "Effects of Forest Bathing on Cardiovascular and Metabolic Parameters in Middle-Aged Males," *Evidence-Based Complementary and Alternative Medicine*, Vol. 2 (2016), pp. 1–7.

10 This was shown by a study that investigated the connection between the living environment of a quarter of a million Americans and their sleep complaints. Those who had access to green spaces were less likely to report poor sleep, and that effect was especially pronounced for men and anyone over the age of sixty-five. See: Diana Grigsby-Toussaint et al., "Sleep Insufficiency and the Natural Environment: Results From the U.S. Behavioral Risk Factor Surveillance System Survey," *Preventive Medicine*, Vol. 78 (September 2015), pp. 78–84.

11 See: Thomas Astell-Burt et al., "Does Access to

Neighbourhood Green Space Promote a Healthy Duration of Sleep? Novel Findings From a Cross-Sectional Study of 259,319 Australians," *BMJ Open*, Vol. 3 (2013).

12   Emi Morita et al., "A Before and After Comparison of the Effects of Forest Walking on the Sleep of a Community-Based Sample of People With Sleep Complaints," *BioPsycho-Social Medicine*, Vol. 5, No. 13 (2011). It is well known that walking reduces stress in general. Exercise reorganizes the brain so that it can better deal with stress. See, for example: T. Schoenfeld et al., "Physical Exercise Prevents Stress-Induced Activation of Granule Neurons and Enhances Local Inhibitory Mechanisms in the Dentate Gyrus," *Journal of Neuroscience*, Vol. 33, No. 18 (2013).

13   This was found by a study carried out in Wisconsin: Benjamin Johnson et al., "Exposure to Neighborhood Green Space and Sleep: Evidence From the Survey of the Health of Wisconsin," *Sleep Health*, Vol. 4, No. 5 (October 2018), pp. 413–419.

14   Ian Alcock et al., "Longitudinal Effects on Mental Health of Moving to Greener and Less Green Urban Areas,"

Environmental Science and Technology, Vol. 48, No. 2 (2014), pp. 1247–1255.

15   For a recent overview of scientific research into the connection between sleep and exposure to green spaces, see: Jong Cheol Shin et al., "Greenspace Exposure and Sleep: A Systematic Review," *Environmental Research*, Vol. 182 (2020).

16   Poor sleep is more common for Indigenous people in Australia and elsewhere. Whatever domain you measure, from sleep duration to fragmented sleep to obstructive sleep apnea (where you stop breathing for a while during sleep), Indigenous people have worse outcomes. According to one study, just under 20 percent of non-Indigenous Australians report sleep disorders, versus almost 35 percent of Aboriginal Australians. See: Garun Hamilton and Simon Joosten, "Sleep Disorders in Indigenous Communities: Time to Close the Gap," *Journal of Clinical Sleep Medicine*, Vol. 11, No. 11 (November 2015), pp. 1255–1256. Sarah Blunden et al., "Sleep Health and Its Implications in First Nation Australians," *The Lancet Western Pacific* (10 February 2022). The percentages are mentioned in "Poor Sleep

More Common for Indigenous People," James Cook University media release (8 January 2022). For Canada, the data are still especially sparse, but a preliminary study found a higher proportion of sleep deprivation among First Nation communities. See: Chandima P. Karunanayake et al., "Duration and Quality of Sleep in 2 Rural Cree First Nation Communities in Saskatchewan, Canada," *Sleep Health*, Vol. 8, No. 2 (April 2022), pp. 146–152.

17 Aboriginal Australians still have the highest rate of children being placed in foster care, Von Senden tells me, and high levels of mental illness. Telephone interview, 20 July 2022. See also: Calla Wahlquist, "'Unfinished Business' of Stolen Generations Puts More Children at Risk," *The Guardian* (22 May 2017).

23:00
Others

1 In *Why Can't We Sleep?*, Darian Leader writes about the social character of sleep. He compares experiments in which people are isolated in order to determine their "natural" sleeping patterns with experiments carried out by King Louis II

of France, who isolated babies from human language. His aim was to determine the "natural language" by seeing if their first words would be Hebrew or Latin.

2 Stephanie Cacioppo et al., "Toward a Neurology of Loneliness," *Psychological Bulletin*, Vol. 140, No. 6 (2014), pp. 1464–1504.

3 This was indicated by a small-scale German study. The couples had 10 percent more REM sleep and their REM sleep was less interrupted when they slept together. See: Henning Drews et al., "Bed-Sharing in Couples Is Associated With Increased and Stabilized REM Sleep and Sleep Stage Synchronization," *Frontiers in Psychiatry* (20 June 2020).

4 See: John Cacioppo, "Do Lonely Days Invade the Nights? Potential Social Modulation of Sleep Efficiency," *Psychological Science*, Vol. 13, No. 4 (July 2002), pp. 384–387. There is a correlation: poor sleep and loneliness often go hand in hand. However, it is not clear whether loneliness *causes* that poor sleep.

5 Johann Hari writes about microarousals and loneliness in *Lost Connections*, p. 78. See also: Lianne Kurina et al.,

"Loneliness Is Associated With Sleep Fragmentation in a Communal Society," *Sleep*, Vol. 34, No. 11 (November 2011), pp. 1519–1526.

6   Eti Ben Simon and Matthew Walker, "Sleep Loss Causes Social Withdrawal and Loneliness," *Nature Communications*, Vol. 9 (2018), p. 3146. Other research shows that married women slept better at night when they had opened up emotionally to their partners during the day. See: Heidi S. Kane et al., "Daily Self-Disclosure and Sleep in Couples," *Health Psychology*, Vol. 33, No. 8 (2014), pp. 813–822.

7   Jen-Hao Chen et al., "Marriage, Relationship Quality, and Sleep Among U.S. Older Adults," *Journal of Health and Social Behavior*, Vol. 56, No. 3 (September 2015), pp. 356–377.

8   See: Robert Meadows and Sara Arber, "Marital Status, Relationship Distress, and Self-Rated Health: What Role for 'Sleep Problems'?," *Journal of Health and Social Behavior*, Vol. 56, No. 3 (2015), pp. 341–355.

9   See: Kerkhof, "Epidemiology of Sleep and Sleep Disorders in the Netherlands."

10   They fell asleep ten minutes sooner on average. Madeline Sprajcer et al., "Sleeping Together: Understanding the Association Between Relationship Type, Sexual Activity, and Sleep," *Sleep Science*, vol. 15 (Jan–March 2022), pp. 80–88.

11   In a large sample of 150,000 Americans, those who have never married report sleep complaints thrice as often as those who are married; those who are divorced had 2.24 times the odds of sleeping poorly as those who were married. M. Grandner et al., "Who Gets the Best Sleep? Ethnic and Socioeconomic Factors Related to Sleep Complaints," *Sleep Medicine*, Vol. 11, No. 5 (May 2010), pp. 470–478.

12   See: Robert Meadows and Sara Arber, "Marital Status, Relationship Distress, and Self-Rated Health," *Journal of Health and Social Behavior*, Vol. 56, No. 3 (2015), pp. 341–355.

13   See: Wendy Troxel et al., "Marital Quality and the Marital Bed: Examining the Covariation Between Relationship Quality and Sleep," *Sleep Medical Review*, Vol. 11, No. 5 (2007), pp. 389–404. The relationship between sleep and loneliness is not simple and may work both ways. Matthew Walker suggests that a lack of sleep makes people lonely, instead of (primarily) vice versa.

Test subjects who were kept awake at night kept a greater distance from others the following day. His hypothesis: the parts of the brain that warn you about people approaching become overactive as a result of a lack of sleep. Other people subsequently also kept a greater distance from the test subject, from which Walker deduces that this distancing is "contagious." "Sleep deprivation can turn us into social lepers," he concluded in an interview with *MarketWatch*. See: Quentin Fottrell, "Nearly Half of Americans Report Feeling Alone," *MarketWatch* (10 October 2018). For the study itself, see: Eti Ben Simon and Matthew Walker, "Sleep Loss Causes Social Withdrawal and Loneliness," *Nature Communications*, Vol. 9, No. 3146 (2018). The consensus seems to be that bad sleep is bad for your relationship, and a bad relationship is bad for your sleep; "sleep problems can be both the cause and the consequence of family conflict." See: Dustin T. Duncan, Ichiro Kawachi, and Susan Redline (ed.), *The Social Epidemiology of Sleep* (Oxford: Oxford University Press, 2019), chapter 12.

14   These figures are taken from the Dutch government's website Volksgezondheid en Zorg.

See: "Eenzaamheid, Cijfers & Context—Meer dan 40 percent van de volwassen bevolking voelt zich eenzaam" (24 September 2020). Those aged eighty-five or above and with a lower level of education are especially lonely. The Statistics Netherlands figures are lower: almost one in ten Dutch people feel very lonely, and more than a quarter feel lonely to some extent. See: "Bijna 1 op de 10 Nederlanders voelde zich sterk eenzaam in 2019," Statistics Netherlands (27 March 2020).

15   See: Brian Resnick, "22 Percent of Millennials Say They Have 'No Friends,'" *Vox* (1 August 2019).

16   This is according to the Canadian Social Survey of 2021, "Loneliness in Canada," Statistics Canada (November 2021).

17   Roughly 28 percent say they feel lonely three or more days a week; fully half feel lonely at least once a week, according to the Australian Loneliness Report (2018).

18   Approximately 14 percent of Brits say they are often or always lonely. See: Tara John, "How the World's First Loneliness Minister Will Tackle 'the Sad Reality of Modern Life,'" *Time* (25 April 2018).

19   The Sleep Foundation website states that "separation anxiety" peaks between eighteen months and three years of age, often leading to a so-called "sleep regression." Eric Suni, "18-Month Sleep Regression," Sleep Foundation (11 March 2022).

20   This connection with (social) insecurity could explain why feelings of loneliness are more likely to affect the sleep of people who have suffered from violence or abuse. A British longitudinal study on twins shows that feelings of loneliness are connected with bad sleep, and that the sleep of people who have been victims of violence or abuse in their youth is particularly strongly impacted when they feel lonely. Perhaps this is because they are quicker to feel unsafe and therefore also stay alert at night. As this relates to research on twins, the researchers are also able to conclude that the effects on sleep are independent of potential genetic susceptibility to sleep problems. See: T. Matthews et al., "Sleeping With One Eye Open: Loneliness and Sleep Quality in Young Adults," *Psychological Medicine*, Vol. 47, No. 12 (September 2017), pp. 2177–2186.

21   Verhaeghe goes into this in more detail in his book *What About Me? The Struggle for Identity in a Market-Based Society*, in the chapter "The New Disorders: Rank and Yank." In it, he refers to figures from the Foundation for Pharmaceutical Statistics from 2011, which show that the use of antidepressants in the Netherlands increased by 230 percent over a period of fifteen years.

22   This is sometimes referred to as "flow." Scientist Mihaly Csikszentmihalyi wrote a famous book about it. See: Mihaly Csikszentmihalyi, *Flow: The Psychology of Optimal Experience* (New York: Harper & Row, 1990).

23   "Flow" sounds delightfully languid, but I think another term better captures the spiritedness to which I refer. The French have the word *élan*, which means the energy of something that moves, an energy that keeps that thing in motion. Élan is akin to momentum, the energy of the activity itself. Élan is also something you can give or receive: you can give an organization "new élan," for example, or you can get that burst of energy yourself from someone or something. Élan is therefore not something that just comes from you yourself, or

your ego, but from what you do or who or what surrounds you.

24　The more materialistic the people, the less often they experience "flow." Why is that? First of all, materialism focuses on increasing your *own* possessions, and that egocentrism doesn't complement "immersing yourself in something different." Secondly, materialism is far removed from your "intrinsic motivation." Intrinsic motivation means that you do things because of the things themselves, because you find them important or because they make you happy. You can often lose yourself in things you do purely due to intrinsic motivation. People who act on the basis of materialism are focused on the outside world. Do I have more or less than others? You buy those expensive jeans and you want that salary because you hope to achieve something *different* through them: status, popularity, etc. You are, in other words, extrinsically motivated. Your satisfaction ought to come from external sources, but often it doesn't come at all. And that is stressful. Your flow is gone. See: Amy Isham et al., "Materialism and the Experience of Flow," *Journal of Happiness Studies* (17 July 2020).

25　See: S. Hershner et al., "Associations Between Transgender Identity, Sleep, Mental Health and Suicidality Among a North American Cohort of College Students," *Nature and Science of Sleep*, Vol. 13 (January 2021), pp. 383–398.

26　The percentages are: 19.3 percent of whites against 43.4 percent of Black Americans, with 37.1 percent of Chinese Americans and 31.5 percent of Latinx Americans sleeping less than six hours per night. Rodrigo Pérez Ortega, "Divided We Sleep," *Science*, Vol. 374, No. 6567 (28 October 2021). Black Americans are also more likely to be long sleepers, which is unhealthy too.

27　See for instance: M.E. Petrov and K.L. Lichstein, "Differences in Sleep Between Black and White Adults: An Update and Future Directions," *Sleep Medicine*, Vol. 18 (February 2016), pp. 74–81.

28　For an overview of research on this topic, see: Dustin T. Duncan, Ichiro Kawachi, and Susan Redline (eds.), *The Social Epidemiology of Sleep* (Oxford: Oxford University Press, 2019), chapter 11. It's interesting to note that both major experiences of discrimination and smaller, chronic everyday aggressions weigh on sleep.

29 Elvira Vedelago, "Parlance: Tricia Hersey," *Postscript* (2021).

30 The "superwoman schema" leads Black American women to sacrifice sleep, as found in the following study: C.L. Woods-Giscombé, "Superwoman Schema: African American Women's Views on Stress, Strength, and Health," *Qualitative Health Research*, Vol. 20, No. 5 (May 2010), pp. 668–683.

31 Vedelago, "Parlance: Tricia Hersey."

32 Ibid.

33 "Tricia Hersey on Rest as Resistance" (transcript), *For the Wild* podcast (5 January 2022).

34 Amina Khan, "How Nap Guru Tricia Hersey Gets It Done," *The Cut* (2020).

35 Vedelago, "Parlance: Tricia Hersey." Jonathan Crary's *24/7* similarly points to capitalism as the beast that devours our sleep.

36 Ibid.

37 "The Nap Ministry Wants You to Know You Are Worthy of Rest," *Here & Now Radio* (21 April 2022).

38 Khan, "How Nap Guru Tricia Hersey Gets It Done."

39 "Tricia Hersey on Rest as Resistance." Hersey's book, *Rest Is Resistance*, wasn't yet out at the time of writing.

00:00
The Weight of Sleep

1 *Walden* is Thoreau's denouncement of modern society. The book opposes the grueling speed of communication and commerce, noise pollution, sensation-seeking reporting, and tight schedules—and this was in 1845. See: Benjamin Reiss, "Happy Birthday to Henry David Thoreau, a Great Sleep Scholar," *Los Angeles Times* (12 July 2017).

2 See: "Sleep and Mental Health," *Harvard Mental Health Letter* (18 March 2019).

3 Two further examples: Matthew Walker, the popular interpreter of the current state of sleep research, gives advice really similar to the above. Make sure your bedroom is cool and dark without any electrical gadgets, move more, etc. His tips are aimed at the "average" sleeper, not the chronic insomniac. He doesn't offer any advice to deal with "real insomnia," for example, if you have already tried his advice to no

avail, as he attributes chronic insomnia to "innate, biological" causes; a chronic lack of sleep suggests a disorder that comes from the person themself, he writes—from which I, suffering from a chronic lack of sleep, derive that nothing can be done about it. The Dutch Brain Foundation offers similar tips to improve the duration and quality of your sleep, from adjusting your bedroom ("make your bed a nice place to sleep") to the way in which you prepare for the night in the evening ("go to bed at the same time each day"). This type of scientifically based advice seeps through to women's magazines, with an extra touch of consumerism: "try aromatherapy" or "natural sleeping remedies," "get a massage." See: Quirine Brouwer, "Moeite met in slaap komen? Déze 20 wetenschappelijke tips kunnen je helpen," Margriet.nl (20 September 2020).

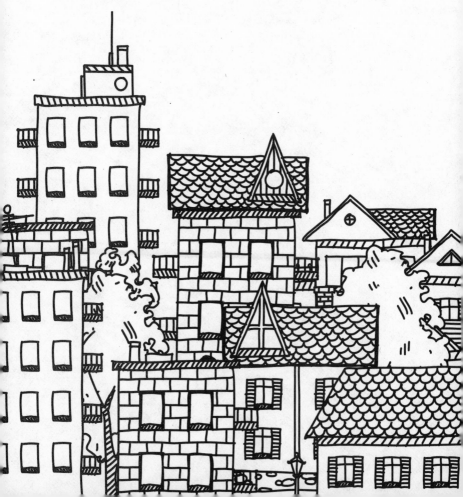

INDEX

A

Aboriginal Australians and Torres Strait Islanders, 167–71, 238n16, 239n17

adenosine, 25–26, 66

adolescents, 99, 142, 203n4, 221n20, 222nn21–22. *See also* children

affects, 115, 116–17, 126, 225n3. *See also* emotions

aggression, 29, 217n3

alertness. *See* hyperarousal; microalertness; microarousals

Ambien (zolpidem), 21, 38, 39, 210n7, 211nn8–9. *See also* sleeping pills

amygdala, 29, 88, 90, 120, 217n3

animals, and sleep, 19–20, 63, 204n6. *See also* birds

antidepressants, 100, 129, 222n24, 227n10

antihistamines, 35

anxiety disorders: author's experience, 42–43; forest bathing and, 167; Hari on, 223n34; increasing prevalence of, 99, 100, 178–79, 222n24; insomnia and, 83–86, 101, 218n8; social context and, 135. *See also* depression; mood

appetite, increased, 207n4

arousal. *See* hyperarousal; microalertness; microarousals

Asclepius, 226n2

Australia: Aboriginal Australians and Torres Strait Islanders, 167–71, 238n16, 239n17; loneliness, 175, 241n17; relationships and sleep, 174; work pace and insomnia, 235n7

autonomous thinking, 111. *See also* unconscious

awake, while sleeping, 61–64

B

Barcelona, 145

Belgium, 234n46

belonging, sense of, 158–61, 176–77

benzodiazepines, 38, 129, 209nn1–2, 210n3, 210n5. *See also* sleeping pills

Beradt, Charlotte, 131–32

Bible, 226n1

biological clock, 66–67, 68, 106–7

birds, 36, 63, 209n1

Black Americans: Black women and "superwomen," 143, 186, 232n34, 244n30; Hersey's Nap Ministry and, 186–87; sleep problems among, 97, 99, 142, 185–86, 220n7, 230n21, 243n26; wealth inequality and, 142, 230n18

blankets, weighted, 174–75

blood alcohol content, 28, 207n1

blue light, 106–7, 225n6

body awareness, 116–17, 226n4

brain: alertness and, 71; dreams and, 120; emotional processing and, 81–82, 83–84, 214n1; hyperarousal and emotional processing, 81–82; limitations of neurological explanation for insomnia, 91;

monitoring using EEG, 54–55, 57,
58; plasticity of, 222n25, 225n8;
sleep deprivation impacts, 28–29,
87–90, 217n3. *See also* hyperarousal
Branson, Richard, 22
Breslau, Naomi, 216n2
Britain. *See* United Kingdom
Buddhism, Tibetan, 226n1
Burton, Robert, 215n2

C
caffeine, 25–26, 207n16
Canada: COVID-19 pandemic and
sleep problems, 100; gender and
insomnia, 142, 231n28; Indigenous
people and sleep problems, 168,
238n16; loneliness, 175; sleeping
pills usage, 38, 210n4; universal
basic income experiment, 144–45,
234n45
cancer, 30, 41, 144, 208n7, 211n9
cannabis, 34–35
capitalism, 178, 186–87, 206n6,
244n35. *See also* productivity
car accidents, 28, 41, 63, 97, 210n4,
212n8
Carnegie, Dale, 24
children, 99, 176, 222n22. *See also*
adolescents
China, 25, 98, 207n14
Chinese Americans, 185, 230n21,
243n26
Churchill, Winston, 22
Cioran, Emil, 77–78, 214n6
circadian rhythm, 66. *See also* clock,
biological
climate change, 136, 227n4
clock, biological, 66–67, 68, 106–7
coffee, 25–26, 207nn15–16
cognitive behavioral therapy, 210n8
coma (vegetative sleep), 60
competition, 178
consciousness, while asleep, 61–64
control, need for, 47
COVID-19 pandemic, 100–101, 131, 136,
144, 151, 223n29, 235n1

Crary, Jonathan, 206n6, 244n35
creativity, 122–23
Csikszentmihalyi, Mihaly, 242n22

D
Dauphin (MB), 144–45
Daylight Savings Time, 28, 207n2
deep sleep. *See* NREM sleep
Denmark, 99
depression: antidepressants, 100, 129,
222n24, 227n10; dreams and, 127;
forest bathing and, 167; gender
nonconforming people and, 184;
Hari on, 223n34, 227n3; increasing
prevalence of, 99, 100, 178–79,
222n24; and insomnia and other
sleep problems, 83–86, 88–91,
215nn2–3, 216n2, 218n8; social
context and, 135. *See also* anxiety
disorders; mood
digital contact, 175
discrimination and racism, 185–87,
243n28
disorders, nature of, 105–6, 223n34
dolphins, 20
Dorsey, Jack, 22
dreams: author's experience, 123–24,
130–31; brain activity during, 120;
as chance by-product of the brain,
120–21; collective dreams, 131–32;
creativity and, 122–23; during deep
sleep, 59; dream rebound effect,
127; emotions and, 121–22, 127;
Freud's dream work theory, 124–25;
listening to and remembering,
128–29, 130; lucid dreams, 129;
as meaningful messages, 119,
226n1; nightmares, 59, 125, 212n4;
physical illness and, 127–28, 226n2;
psychological problems and,
127; tips for increasing, 129–30;
unconscious and, 125–26. *See also*
REM sleep
Dutch Brain Foundation, 244n3

E

earthworms, 20
Edison, Thomas, 23–24
education, 141, 144, 229nn13–15, 233n41, 241n14
ego-building: alternatives to, 180–84; insomnia from, 179–80
élan, 242n23. *See also* flow
electroencephalogram (EEG), 53–55, 57, 58
elephant seals, 19
emotions: affects, 115, 116–17, 126, 225n3; approach to, 91–92; dreams and, 121–22, 127; emotional dysregulation, 88; incomplete processing of, 80–82, 83–84, 214n1; sleep deprivation and, 29, 89, 217n3; sleep problems and, 101, 109, 223nn31–32; tips for discovering, 116–17; as unconscious, 113–15. *See also* anxiety disorders; depression; mood
employment, 236n11. *See also* night shift; unemployment
endowment effect, 163, 164
England. *See* United Kingdom
enjoyment, 182–83
environment. *See* place
epidemiological research, 224n2
eszopiclone (Lunesta), 211n8. *See also* sleeping pills
ethnicity. *See* race
exercise, 238n12

F

fight-or-flight response. *See* sympathetic nervous system
Finland, 99
FIRE (Financial Independence, Retire Early) movement, 146–47, 234n48
fish, 63
Fitbit, 140
flamingos, 19
flow, 182, 242nn22–23, 243n24
Ford, Tom, 22
forest bathing, 166–67, 237n10
France, 97, 235n6

Freud, Sigmund, 111, 119, 120–21, 124–25, 126–27
frugality, 145–46, 147–48, 148–50

G

GABA, 39
gadgets, sleep, 139–40, 228n6
gender, 97, 142–43, 184, 219n4, 230nn23–25, 231nn27–29, 232n34
gender nonconforming people, 184, 230n23
genes, 67–68, 84–85, 215n1
ghrelin, 207n4
Gioia, Dana: "Insomnia," 214n4, 232n38
good intentions, 156
Great Britain. *See* United Kingdom
green spaces, 166–67, 237n10
group edge effect, 36, 209n1
Guinness World Records, 30

H

happiness, 182–84, 199
Hari, Johann: *Lost Connections*, 223n34, 227n3
Harvard Medical School, 197
health, physical, 30, 127–28, 226n2
here and now, 157–58
Hersey, Tricia, 186–87
Herzberg, Judith: "The Way," 110
hippocampus, 29, 88, 89, 90, 120
Hippocrates, 119
Hispanic/Latinx people, 142, 185, 230n21, 243n26
homeostasis, 66–67, 68
hormones: appetite and, 207n4; melatonin, 99, 106–7, 221n18
hunter-gatherers, 205n3
Hutterites, 173
hyperarousal: author's experience as a writer, 75–77; daytime alertness among insomniacs, 73–75; emotional processing and, 80–82; insomnia from, 70–72; limitations as an explanation, 108; sleep gadgets and, 140; value of despite

insomnia, 77–79, 214n4, 214nn6–7; weightlessness sensation, 189
hypersomnia, 85, 215n3

I

Iceland, 99
IKEA effect, 162–64
illness, physical, 30, 127–28, 226n2
implicit thinking, 111. *See also* unconscious
income: health and, 232n37; sleep problems and, 141, 143, 223n30, 229n11, 232n36; universal basic income, 144–45, 234n45. *See also* money
Indigenous people, 168, 238n16. *See also* Aboriginal Australians and Torres Strait Islanders
individualism, 178–79. *See also* ego-building
Industrial Revolution, 23, 105–6
insomnia: animals and, 204n6; approach to, 14–15, 48–49, 102, 197–200; author's journey with, 12–13, 14–15, 20, 32–36, 37–38, 42–43, 45–46, 72, 102, 108, 140–41, 191–93, 218n9; biological and scientific approaches to, 91, 95–96, 101, 104–5, 107, 216nn5–6, 218n3; biological clock and, 66–67, 68, 106–7; as call to action, 198–99; common advice for, 95–96, 197–98, 244n3; COVID-19 pandemic and, 100–101, 223n29; diagnostic criteria, 203n5; effects of sleep deprivation, 27–30, 207nn2–4, 208n7, 208n9, 212n8; genes and, 67–68, 215n1; homeostasis and, 66–67, 68; hyperarousal and, 70–72; increase and prevalence, 20, 96–97, 98–99, 203nn3–5, 218nn1–2, 220n11, 220n13, 221n18; vs. letting go (surrendering), 47–48, 181–84; meaning of life and, 117–18, 178; mood and, 87–91; overlap with anxiety and depression, 83–86, 215n3, 216n2, 218n8, 223n34; rebound insomnia, 40; vs. sleep state misperception, 52; social context and, 135–37; unconscious and, 116. *See also* hyperarousal; money; others; place; sleep problems; time
intentions, good, 156
Inuit: "Utitia'q's Song," 214n7
Islam, 226n1

J

Japan, 25, 167
jet lag, 66

K

Kafka, Franz, 189
Kasius, Kristel, 152

L

Lancel, Marieke, 217n3
latent awareness, 64
Latinx/Hispanic people, 142, 185, 230n21, 243n26
Leader, Darian, 104, 125–26, 239n1
learn, capacity to, 29
leptin, 207n4
letting go (surrendering), 47–48, 181–84
life, meaning of, 117–18, 178
light: blue light, 106–7, 225n6; light pollution, 13
living costs, 147–48, 234n46
loneliness, 172–73, 175, 177, 239n4, 240n13, 241n13, 241nn17–18, 242n20
Louis II (French king), 239n1
lucid dreams, 129
Lunesta (eszopiclone), 211n8. *See also* sleeping pills

M

marijuana, 34–35
materialism, 182, 243n24
McCartney, Paul, 113
medication: antidepressants, 100, 129,

222n24, 227n10; antihistamines,
35; sleeping pills, 37–41, 129, 140–
41, 209nn1–2, 210nn3–5, 210n7,
211nn8–9
Meerlo, Peter, 87–90, 216n2, 217n3
melancholy, 85, 215n2. *See also*
depression
melatonin, 99, 106–7, 221n18
Mendeleev, Dmitri, 113
mental health, and social context,
135, 227nn1–3. *See also* anxiety
disorders; depression
Menzis, 31
mere exposure effect, 163
micro-alertness, 65
microarousals, 173
microsleep, 64
Milky Way, 11–12, 13
money: commercialization of sleep,
138–40, 228nn2–3, 228n6;
frugality and time, 145–50, 194–95;
income and sleep problems, 141,
143, 223n30, 229n11, 232n36; living
costs, 147–48, 234n46; universal
basic income, 144–45, 234n45;
wealth inequality and race, 141–42,
230n18
mood, 87–91. *See also* anxiety
disorders; depression
Morpheus, 45
Mr. Money Mustache, 146–47
Musk, Elon, 21, 31

N
Nabokov, Vladimir, 77
Nap Ministry, 187
Napoleon, 22
naps, 25, 187, 207n14
narcolepsy, 213n2
nature, and forest bathing, 166–67,
237n10
Netherlands: antidepressants, 227n10;
education and insomnia, 141,
229n14; gender and insomnia, 142;
income and insomnia, 141, 229n11;
living costs, 234n46; loneliness,

175, 241n13; night shift and shift
work, 233n41; prevalence of
insomnia, 24, 98, 99, 203n3, 218n2,
222n23; race and insomnia, 97,
219n5; sleep and relationships, 174;
sleeping pills, 38; time pressure and
insomnia, 152, 235n2
nightmares, 59, 125, 212n4. *See also*
dreams
night shift, 30, 144, 232n40, 233n41
nocturnal panic, 125–26
non-binary people, 184, 230n23
non-fearful panic attack, 113–14
noradrenaline, 75, 80, 81–82, 87, 122,
215n4
Norway, 98, 220n11
NREM sleep (deep sleep): alertness
while asleep and, 64;
characteristics and phases, 57–58,
59–60, 212n2, 212n4; depression
and, 215n3; race and, 142. *See also*
REM sleep

O
orgasms, 183
others: flow and, 182, 242nn22–23,
243n24; vs. individualism and ego-
building, 178–80; vs. loneliness,
172–73, 175, 177, 239n4, 240n13,
241n13, 241nn17–18, 242n20;
sense of (in)security from, 176–77,
242n20; sense of threat from, 184–
87; sleep and, 172–74, 239n1, 239n3,
240n6, 240n10–11; surrendering to,
47–48, 181–84; weight of, 195–96
otters, 19
oxazepam, 38, 209n1. *See also* sleeping
pills

P
pain, 92, 218n9
panic, nocturnal, 125–26
panic attack, non-fearful, 113–14
paradoxical insomnia (sleep state
misperception), 52, 212n1
paradoxical sleep, 57

parasomnias, 60, 212n2
Perec, Georges: *A Man Asleep*, 206n6
periodic limb movement disorder, 213n2
place: Aboriginal Australians and, 167–71; author's move to Burgundian village, 148, 161–62, 164–65, 190–91, 192–93, 195–96; challenges being present, 157–58; disconnection from, 161; forest bathing, 166–67, 237n10; IKEA effect, 162–64; sense of belonging, 158–61; urban environments, 165–66; weight of, 196–97
Plato, 205n4
pleasure, 183–84
Pokémon Go, 228n4
Pokémon Sleep, 138–39
post-traumatic stress disorder (PTSD), 215n4, 223n29
prefrontal cortex, 28, 29, 114, 217n3
present, being, 157–58
productivity, 27, 30–31, 208n9. *See also* capitalism
purpose, sense of, 117–18, 178

Q
Quran, 226n1

R
race: sleep problems and, 97, 142, 219nn5–6, 220n7, 230n21, 243n26; wealth inequality and, 141–42, 230n18, 232n34
racism and discrimination, 185–87, 243n28
Raskind, Murray, 215n4
rats, 88–89, 90, 204n6, 217n4
rebound insomnia, 40
relationships. *See* others
relaxation, 46, 183. *See also* surrendering
REM sleep (dream sleep): barriers to, 129–30; brain activity during, 120; characteristics and phases, 56–57, 212n1; depression and, 215n3;

effects from deprivation, 121; emotional processing and, 80–81, 83; hyperarousal and, 70; PTSD and, 215n4. *See also* dreams; NREM sleep
reset, 35, 191–92
restless legs syndrome, 67
Robb, Alice, 127
romantic relationships, 173–74, 239n3, 240n6, 240nn10–11

S
Sacks, Oliver, 128
Sandman, 45
scientific methods, 103–5, 216n5, 224n2
scientism, 224n1
security, sense of, 176–77, 242n20. *See also* threat, sense of
sedatives, 37–41, 129, 140–41, 209nn1–2, 210nn3–5, 210nn7–8, 211n9
self. *See* ego-building
Seoul, 158
separation anxiety, 176, 242n19
serotonin, 88–89
Shakespeare, William: *Henry IV, Part 2*, 205n4
Shelley, Mary, 113
shift work disorder, 232n40. *See also* night shift
sleep: by animals, 19–20, 63, 204n6; author's childhood experiences, 44–45; capitalism and, 178, 186–87, 206n6, 244n35; coffee and, 25–26; commercialization of, 138–40, 228nn2–3, 228n6; decline of, 24–25; denigration of, 21–22, 23–24, 77, 205n4; effects of sleep deprivation, 27–30, 207nn2–4, 208n7, 208n9, 212n8; emotional processing during, 80–82, 83–84, 214n1; as enemy to defeat, 46–47; letting go (surrendering) for, 47–48, 181–84; microsleep, 63; monitoring using EEG, 53–55, 57, 58; mood and, 87–91; mysteriousness of, 53; in premodern times, 22–23,

105–6, 205n3; productivity and, 27, 30–31, 208n9; research on, 221n15; wakefulness during, 61–64. *See also* insomnia; money; NREM sleep; others; place; REM sleep; sleep problems; time

sleep apnea, 67, 213n2

sleep cycle, 58–59

sleeper cars, on trains, 44–45

sleep graphs, 53–55, 57, 58

sleep hygiene, 32–34, 68, 197, 200

sleeping pills, 37–41, 129, 140–41, 209nn1–2, 210nn3–5, 210nn7–8, 211n9

sleeping sickness, 128

sleep maintenance disorder, 105–6

sleep problems: in adolescents and children, 99, 142, 203n4, 221n20, 222nn21–22; and anxiety and depression, 83–86, 88–91, 215nn2–3, 216n2, 218n8; climate crisis and, 227n4; discrimination and, 185–87, 243n28; education and, 141, 144, 229nn14–15; emotions and, 101, 109, 223nn31–32; gender and, 97, 142–43, 184, 219n4, 230nn23–25, 231nn27–29; income and, 141, 143, 229n11, 232n36; vs. lack of sleep, 213n1; race and, 97, 142, 219nn5–6, 220n7, 230n21, 243n26; time pressure and, 151–53, 235nn6–7, 236n8; use of term, 213n2. *See also* insomnia

sleep regression, 242n19

sleep state misperception (paradoxical insomnia), 52, 212n1

sleep therapy, 43–44, 46–48

smartphones, 107, 154, 158, 183, 225n7, 237n1

socioeconomic inequality: education and, 141, 144, 229nn13–15, 233n41, 241n14; gender and, 97, 142–43, 184, 219n4, 230nn23–25, 231nn27–29, 232n34; income and sleep problems, 141, 143, 223n30, 229n11, 232n36; race and sleep problems, 97, 142, 219nn5–6,

220n7, 230n21, 243n26; race and wealth inequality, 141–42, 230n18, 232n34; unemployment and, 97–98, 144, 233n43

Somnox, 140

Spain, 25

spiders, 20

SSRIS, 209n2. *See also* sleeping pills

Stickgold, Robert, 122–23, 225n2

stress system (sympathetic nervous system), 71–72, 95, 108, 213n2. *See also* hyperarousal

Sturt, George: *Change in the Village*, 158–61, 237n4

subconscious. *See* unconscious

suicide, 85, 127, 222n24

sunrise alarm (wake-up light), 72

surrendering (letting go), 47–48, 181–84

Sweden, 99

sympathetic nervous system (stress system), 71–72, 95, 108, 213n2. *See also* hyperarousal

T

teenagers. *See* adolescents

temazepam, 37–38, 39, 209n1. *See also* sleeping pills

therapy: author's experience with sleep therapy, 43–44, 46–48; cognitive behavioral therapy, 210n8; for discovering unconscious, 117

Thoreau, Henry David, 193; *Walden*, 193, 244n1

threat, sense of, 184–87. *See also* security, sense of

Tibetan Buddhism, 226n1

time: COVID-19 pandemic and, 151, 235n1; free time between tasks, 153–55, 195; frugality and, 145–50, 194–95; time banks, 234n49; time pressure and sleep problems, 151–53, 235nn6–7, 236n8; tips for finding, 155–56

traffic accidents, 28, 41, 63, 97, 210n4, 212n8

trains, sleeper cars, 44–45
transgender people, 184, 230n23
trauma, 83. *See also* post-traumatic
  stress disorder (PTSD)
Trump, Donald, 22

U

unconscious: author's experience,
  109; brain activity and, 111–12;
  conscious thinking and, 112–13;
  dreams and, 125–26; emotion
  and, 113–15; insomnia and, 116;
  subconscious thinking, 110–11; tips
  for discovering, 116–17
unemployment, 97–98, 144, 233n43
United Kingdom: anxiety disorders,
  222n24; education and sleep
  problems, 141; gender inequalities,
  143, 231n29; green spaces and
  mental health, 167; loneliness, 175,
  241n18; prevalence of insomnia,
  25, 98, 99; sleeping pills, 210n5;
  smartphone use, 225n7

United Nations, 135, 227n2
United States of America: education
  inequalities, 141, 229n13, 229n15;
  gender inequalities, 143, 219n4;
  income inequalities, 141; loneliness,
  175; mental health issues, 222n24;
  prevalence of insomnia, 24–25,
  98–99, 206n11, 221n18; race
  inequalities, 97, 142, 143, 219n6,
  220n7, 230n21; relationships and
  sleep, 174, 240n11; sleeping pills, 38
universal basic income, 144–45,
  234n45
urban environments, 165–66
"Utitia'q's Song," 214n7

V

Van der Helm, Els, 27–30, 73, 208n9
Van Someren, Eus: on comas
  (vegetative sleep), 60; on dreaming,
  59; on electroencephalograms (EEGs),
  53–54; on genetics, 67–68, 84–85;
  on hyperarousal, 73–75, 80, 81–82;
  on latent awareness, 64; on overlap
  between anxiety, depression, and

insomnia, 83, 84–85, 86; on REM
sleep, 57, 87; on sleep gadgets, 140;
on sleeping pills, 39
vegetative sleep (coma), 60
Verhaeghe, Paul: on enjoyment
and surrender, 180–81, 182–83;
formula for sleep, 184; on Freud's
dream work theory, 125; on
individualism and ego-building,
178–80; on scientism, 224n1; on
sense of security, 176–77; on social
context of mental health, 227n3;
on unconscious emotion, 113–14,
115, 116, 225n3; on unconscious
thinking, 110–11, 112–13
Verkooijen, Sanne, 43–44, 47–48, 71
Von Senden, Roslyn, 167–71, 239n17

W

wakefulness, while sleeping, 61–64
wake-up light (sunrise alarm), 72
Walker, Matthew: advice for sleep,
244n3; on coffee, 25, 207n15;
on gender, 219n4, 230n24; on
insomnia, 32, 52, 95, 96, 101,
140, 218n3, 223n32; on loneliness,
240n13; on NREM sleep, 58; on
sleep deprivation effects, 208n7,
212n8; on sleep gadgets, 228n6; on
sleeping pills, 39, 211n9; on stress
system, 71
walking, 226n4, 238n12
weight: author's experience being
weighed down, 45–46, 174–75,
189–90; comparison to roots,
193–94; of others, 195–96; of place,
196–97; of time, 194–95; weighted
blankets, 174–75; weightlessness
sensation, 189
willpower, 65
work, type of, 236n11
World Health Organization (WHO), 23,
24, 99, 135, 144, 222n24
worry, 101. *See also* anxiety disorders

Z

Z-drugs, 38, 209n2, 210n5. *See also*
sleeping pills
zolpidem (Ambien), 21, 38, 39, 210n7,
211nn8–9. *See also* sleeping pills
zopiclone, 39, 209n1, 210n7.
See also sleeping pills

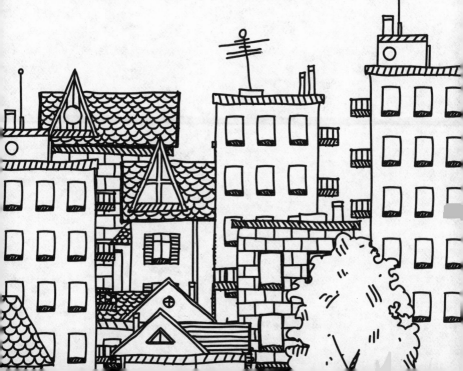